Nursing and Midwifery Portfolios

Nursing and Midwifery Portfolios

Evidence of Continuing Competence, 2e

Kate Andre

Marie Heartfield

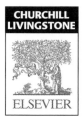

CHURCHILL
LIVINGSTONE

ELSEVIER

Sydney Edinburgh London New York Philadelphia St Louis Toronto

Churchill Livingstone
is an imprint of Elsevier

Elsevier Australia. ACN 001 002 357
(a division of Reed International Books Australia Pty Ltd)
Tower 1, 475 Victoria Avenue, Chatswood, NSW 2067

National Library of Australia Cataloguing-in-Publication Data

Author:	Andre, Kate.
Title:	Nursing and midwifery portfolios: evidence of continuing competence / Kate Andre and Marie Heartfield.
Edition:	2nd ed.
ISBN:	978-0-7295-4078-0 (pbk.)
Subjects:	Employment portfolios—Australia. Employment portfolios—New Zealand.
	Nursing—Standards—Australia. Nursing—Standards—New Zealand.
	Midwifery—Standards—Australia. Midwifery—Standards—New Zealand.

Other Authors/Contributors: Heartfield, Marie.
Dewey Number: 610.730690994

Publisher: Libby Houston
Developmental Editor: Elizabeth Coady
Publishing Services Manager: Helena Klijn
Project Coordinators: Geraldine Minto and Karthikeyan Murthy
Edited by Stephanie Pickering
Proofread by Annette Musker
Illustrations by Shaun Jury
Cover design by Lisa Petroff
Index by Robert Swanson
Typeset by TNQ Books and Journals PVT. Ltd.
Printed by 1010 Printing International Ltd.

Contents

Contents

Foreword

We, in the professions of nursing and midwifery, owe a debt of gratitude to Kate Andre and Marie Heartfield for this most timely book. In our pre- or post-registration professional lives, we are being asked to construct professional portfolios and to provide evidence of our continuing competence for the purposes of education, employment or registration. There is much agreement as to the need for being able to provide the portfolios, but little knowledge of just how to go about it.

Since the regulatory authorities in both Australia and New Zealand started including a need for evidence of continuing competence in their registration processes, much concern has been expressed about just what this means and there is complete confusion as to how to go about providing it. Nurses and midwives have a legal and ethical responsibility to demonstrate their competence to practise, but the means by which this is to be achieved is relatively new to many.

In this book, Marie and Kate have provided us with an elegant, accessible and extensively referenced guide through the process. We are introduced here to an understanding of what a portfolio is, what it is used for, methods of design, management and compilation, but most importantly, the reflective skills needed for a process that captures our deep and transformational learning. The book concludes with our being taken full circle in our learning and guides us through the process of evaluating a portfolio, whether for self-assessment or for assessing others.

I strongly recommend this book and only wish it had been written many years ago so that my office shelves would be less full of detritus and my evidence of professional development less chaotic. Marie and Kate, on behalf of my colleague nurses and midwives in Australia and New Zealand, thank you.

Professor Jill White AM, RN, RM, MEd, PhD

Dean, Faculty of Nursing & Midwifery, University of Sydney
Chair, Australian Nursing and Midwifery Accreditation Council (ANMAC)
Deputy Chair, Council of Deans of Nursing, Australia and New Zealand
(CDNM)

Preface

Portfolios are common in university education as a technique through which to learn reflective analysis skills and demonstrate learning. They are increasingly used by midwives and nurses as a tool to guide the review of professional practice. The benefits for nurses and midwives of reviewing professional practice and demonstrating learning is to direct continuing professional development, learning and career planning and communicate professional achievements.

This book will help you to understand the drivers and benefits of portfolios and how to design and evaluate a quality portfolio. Your ability to do this will be assisted by understanding the relationship between professional portfolios and the regulatory requirements of self-declaration and practising in accordance with professional competency standards. Different styles are presented including electronic portfolios and their use for educational and regulatory purposes, as well as professional development and planning. The concepts of designing a portfolio for a specific purpose and the use of quality evidence are the central tenets of this book. Where appropriate, supporting materials have been drawn from a range of Australian, New Zealand and international sources. In addition to providing direction on how to design your own professional portfolio, this book contains information about how to evaluate and assess portfolios developed by others.

Because portfolios are widely used in the educational and professional settings, this book has relevance to a broad audience, from nursing and midwifery students through to clinical experts and health administrators. Primarily this book is for individuals intending to develop their own portfolios; however, it has been written in a manner that is accessible to a wider group including students undertaking other practice-based health science studies. In the first instance, readers may wish to peruse this book to gain a basic understanding of portfolios, including how different approaches are used for different purposes, and to gain a sense of the basic process of developing a portfolio. Much of the content that will assist in this is contained in Chapters 1, 2 and 3. Chapters 4 and 5 provide greater detail about understanding your purpose for developing a portfolio, including assembling components and developing an overall argument. Chapter 6 addresses the assessment of portfolios developed by others and the use of portfolios for career planning. This final chapter also has relevance to those assembling their own portfolio, for it is through this wider perspective that a complete understanding of a quality portfolio may be gained.

Each chapter of this book starts with either key questions that will be explored in the chapter or situations that may motivate readers to learn more about portfolios. The chapters are as follows:

Chapter 1. Professional practice and portfolios: Why do I need a professional portfolio?

This chapter assists the reader to understand the concept of portfolios and their use in self-regulation and professional regulation. The relationship between international (e.g. International Council of Nurses), national (e.g. Australian Nursing and Midwifery Council) and broader generic competencies (e.g. university graduate qualities) is used to illustrate the potential for portfolios to guide the review of professional practice.

Chapter 2. Portfolio styles and models

Portfolios can be used to direct learning, communicate competence and help plan a career. This chapter is designed to enable the reader to appreciate the range of portfolio styles and models and identify the need for, and benefits of, specific models to address individual needs. Having examined the purpose for their own portfolio, the reader is introduced to a range of pragmatic issues associated with accumulating and compiling evidence of learning and competence.

Chapter 3. Reflection and reflective practice

The purpose of this chapter is to assist the reader in understanding and applying reflection techniques in professional development, learning and portfolio use. The meanings and uses of the concept of reflection, and their application to the development of portfolios for nurses, midwives and other health professionals is examined. Specific applications for accomplishing and demonstrating the application and use of reflective skills as a professional achievement are also included.

Chapter 4. Evidence: What do I have and what do I need?

The aim of this chapter is to help the reader to understand the notion of evidence of competent practice and the types, sources and quality of evidence that will support their claims of competence. The reader is guided through a process of identifying existing evidence and generating new evidence of their performance outcomes.

Chapter 5. Compiling your portfolio

This chapter helps the reader to develop and assemble a portfolio. The chapter will show the reader how to put together the various parts of a portfolio so that its intent — to produce an account that demonstrates and evaluates progress towards learning and/or professional competence — is achieved.

Chapter 6. Portfolio evaluation and assessment

A quality portfolio is judged through demonstrated proficiency in selecting, structuring and justifying the requisite evidence. This chapter provides an overview of the basic principles of assessment applied to portfolios and is intended not only for the portfolio developer to assess their portfolio development but also as an introduction for those considering a role as an assessor of portfolios for educational and regulatory purposes. The material also provides an alternative perspective to those submitting their portfolio for assessment.

About the authors

Kate Andre RN, RM, BN, MN, PhD, FRCNA

Kate Andre is Associate Professor of Nursing Education within the School of Nursing Midwifery and Post Graduate Medicine at Edith Cowan University in Western Australia. Kate's PhD research, teaching, publications and consultancy activities are in the area of competency assessment and curriculum design for nurses. Kate has had considerable experience in the implementation and assessment of portfolios, including as: an advisor for the selection and implementation of a University-wide e-portfolio platform (UniSA); a convenor for Nurse Practitioner assessment panels (NMBSA); and a member of a University research team in the use of e-portfolios.

Marie Heartfield RN, BN(Ed), MNS, PhD, FRCNA

Dr Marie Heartfield is Senior Lecturer in the School of Nursing and Midwifery at the University of South Australia. Marie has been involved in a wide range of nursing and healthcare research and education at state, national and international levels, and has taught nurses, midwives and allied health professionals in a range of tertiary undergraduate, graduate and professional programmes since 1989. Other teaching and learning contributions include curricula review and advisory roles, and development of educational policy and national health professional education guidelines. Marie has also been a joint leader in a number of national research projects to review nursing roles and develop core and specialised competency standards.

Reviewers List

Lynette Bowen RN, MN, BEd, Dip. Teach
Lecturer, School of Nursing & Midwifery, University of Newcastle

Carol Crevacore RN, Bachelor Nursing, GCTT
First Year Coordinator, Lecturer in Nursing Edith Cowan University

Lyn Croxon Lecturer, BN
Course Coordinator, School of Nursing, Midwifery & Indigenous Health, Charles Sturt University

Jan M. Sayers RN, Grad. Dip. Ad.Ed., M.A. (Educational Administration)
Director of Learning & Teaching / Lecturer, School of Nursing & Midwifery, University of Western Sydney

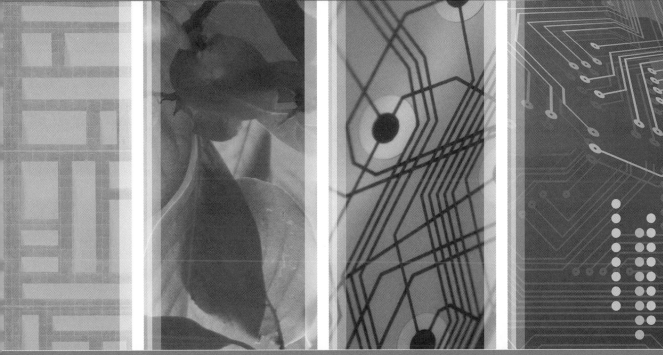

CHAPTER 1

Professional practice and portfolios: Why do I need a professional portfolio?

Introduction

- Your education or training course has assessments that require portfolio-related activities.
- Your nursing or midwifery registration requires you to make a statement about your competence to practise in line with standards of continuing professional development.
- Your induction into a new job highlights an employment obligation to set and report against individual performance goals.
- Your success as a nurse or midwife will need a plan for successful career and work—life balance.

The above situations are common to most nurses and midwives at some stage in their careers. They highlight the aim of this book which is to guide nurses, midwives and other health professionals in understanding how to

Nursing and Midwifery Portfolios. DOI: 10.1016/B978-0-7295-4078-0.10001-8
Copyright © 2011, Elsevier Australia.

develop and present a portfolio that demonstrates their professional efforts, progress and achievements. The book is written for students of both nursing or midwifery as well as for those already practising in these professions and will have relevance for other health professionals.

This first chapter outlines why it is important to know about professional portfolios and how they can be used to provide information that can be useful for your own consideration or for the purposes of others such as

- nursing and midwifery regulatory authorities: to demonstrate your eligibility for initial registration as well as accountability for continuing professional development and continuing registration
- educational providers: to pass a course or programme or apply for recognition of prior learning
- employers: to gain employment or promotion
- professional organisations: for accreditation and/or credential purposes.

As nurses and midwives, we bring together the knowledge and evidence from our own and a range of other disciplines that we use to improve the health experiences of the people in our care. Portfolios provide a way to bring together that knowledge and evidence to communicate to others learning and development as well as a current level of achievement or competency.

Creating a professional portfolio involves an individual examining their existing practice against appropriate expectations or standards (be they personal or professional). The idea is that this process may highlight potential areas for improvement, hence a learning or career plan for continuing professional development. Improved or higher standards of practice open the way for new opportunities, professional and career development.

The obligations of the health workforce and therefore nurses and midwives are complex. As discussed in more detail later in this chapter, nurses and midwives have legal and moral obligations as members of their professions and as individuals. In addition to this the external pressures on them and other healthcare professionals to demonstrate the appropriateness of their clinical and professional decisions have increased considerably. Since the World Health Organization launch in October 2004 of a World Alliance for Patient Safety most countries, including Australia and New Zealand, have established a range of national healthcare safety and quality mechanisms with the clear message that professional competence and ongoing education impact directly on patient safety (Australian Institute of Health and Welfare 2006, Australian Commission on Safety and Quality in Healthcare 2006, Briant et al 2001). The demands on health systems and services directly impact on the health workforce and its training and service delivery. In Australia, health consumer expectations are high and come from our history of being well served by a quality health system to which we have ready and timely access (National Health Workforce Taskforce 2009). For healthcare students and practitioners this translates to the clear need for skills in understanding, generating and using the evidence that communicates how their practice meets the necessary standards of professional responsibility and accountability. This book will examine the forms that such evidence can take as well as the role of skills such as reflection in producing the evidence and the argument for competency.

Nurses and midwives, as healthcare practitioners, have significant responsibilities in providing health interventions and protecting patients from the effects of illness, disability and infirmity. They are not able to go about practice in routine ways; 'the way they always have' or 'because that is how things are done in this health agency'. A significant and continuing challenge for all healthcare practitioners is to stay informed about the knowledge developments and recommended practice changes relevant to their field and role. This is particularly important as healthcare becomes increasingly complex due to an ageing population, increasing shifts to public health, relatively rapid changes in client conditions and expectations, technology, pharmacology, health systems and practitioner roles. All healthcare practitioners have obligations to improve quality and manage threats to client safety. The best available evidence, in whatever form, is necessary as a foundation for all health practitioner actions. The only effective way to manage this expectation is to be continuously learning. Nurses and midwives in Australia and New Zealand are required to demonstrate their continuing professional development as a condition of their registration to practise. Portfolios have a long and reliable history as a useful way to demonstrate learning and therefore progressive achievement of competency.

As a first step in learning about portfolios and gaining confidence to create or refine one, the following discussion outlines portfolios in their various forms and the main reasons for their use in nursing and midwifery.

Summary points

· The purpose of this book is to provide a depth of understanding about why portfolios can support nurses, midwives and other health professionals to develop and extend their practice and careers.
· Nurses, midwives and many other health professionals in Australia and New Zealand have legal and moral obligations to demonstrate understanding and evidence of their level of competency to practise.

What is a portfolio?

The word 'portfolio' is used in various ways depending on the context of use. In a political or organisational sense a portfolio shows an allocation of responsibilities. In education a portfolio is usually a collection of information that informs the demonstration of learning that has occurred for an individual in a specific course or programme of studies. A professional portfolio is a structured collection of different types of information and evidence that show an individual's continuing professional development activities and experiences, competencies, and professional achievements and goals. It is both a repository of detail and a means by which the portfolio author or developer acquires and develops skills in reflective analysis and communication whether this is through written or computer-mediated formats such as e-portfolios.

Like a scrapbook that stores and communicates past events and memories, a portfolio is also a collection of documents, certificates, photos and other artefacts collected over your working life. However, a portfolio to be created and used for professional purposes is more than just a collection of artefacts. It takes its shape as a professional portfolio through the reflections and connections that are built by the portfolio author or developer. Connections are the links between the actual experiences, practices, thought and ideas with the relevant or necessary frameworks, standards, tools or expectations of the individual nurse or midwife and their profession. These connections are created and described by the individual portfolio author most commonly through reflective thinking and analysis. The frameworks, standards, tools or expectations that might shape portfolio connections could be standards such as competency or continuing professional development standards as endorsed by the Nursing and Midwifery Board of Australia or the Nursing Council of New Zealand or the requirements of a particular assignment.

The reflective process of examining current practice across personal, professional, organisational, regulatory and social dimensions provides the insights needed to produce a record of past growth and the likelihood of continued growth. This provides a basis from which to demonstrate the capacity to contribute competently to nursing and/or midwifery and healthcare. A portfolio demonstrates thinking and reasoning and in this sense is an argument. The term argument may seem a strange one to use to some readers and is not commonly used in nursing and midwifery literature. 'Argue' means to give reasons or cite evidence in support of an idea, action or theory, normally done to get others to share your point of view (Oxford Dictionary of English, 2nd edn 2005). An argument is identifiable by a logical or quasi logical sequence of ideas supported by evidence (Andrew 2010) with the important addition of a clear outcome or conclusion.

An effective professional portfolio not only includes description of experiences and practice but links this to the relevant nursing or midwifery knowledge to produce an argument about the level of competence or learning that has been achieved. The portfolio outlines why the claim is legitimate and can be accepted as valid in meeting the required expectations. This type of portfolio applies nursing or midwifery knowledge to the practice of nursing or midwifery for the individual in their particular context or circumstances.

There are many issues that have shaped the increased use of professional portfolios in nursing and midwifery and the main ones are discussed later in this chapter. Variations on what a portfolio looks like, how it is used or why it is needed are all influenced by who is seeking what information and for what purpose. Although the concept of evidence will be discussed in detail in Chapter 3, it is important to understand that this means different things to different people. Evidence means a support or verification, yet it can also be interpreted as proof. Evidence may be produced by others (such as a certificate of achievement) or produced by the individual (such as through reflective thinking).

The evidence necessary to acquire and demonstrate competence or learning is complex, takes time and varies depending on practice context, education and experience. A professional portfolio is a medium that contains documents such as care plans, employer statements and certificates of attendance at courses, glued together through processes of reflective analysis to create a forward looking document that demonstrates achievements and goals competent nursing and midwifery practice.

Summary points

·   A professional portfolio is a collection of resources: a repository and a means through which to develop skills in reflective analysis and communication, whether through written or computer-mediated formats.
·   Portfolios help to demonstrate and support the following:
  ·   individual reflective thinking and writing processes
  ·   employment, education and professional and personal development
  ·   performance based on analysis of previous and current practice, competence based on analysis of previous and current knowledge, skills and experiences
  ·   application of knowledge to practise though an understanding of how context may shape competency and practice
  ·   learning based on knowledge acquisition and skill development
  ·   future goals and career direction based on consideration and analysis of the previous two points.

Activity: Professional roles

As a first step in building a portfolio write a brief description of what your profession does or what your professional role is. Write this for someone who would not already know about nursing or midwifery or would have a layperson's understanding.

You may wish to keep your answers at hand so that you can review them as your portfolio develops.

Forms of portfolios

Portfolios can take many forms. Other chapters in this book will explore these in more detail though for now we start from the idea of a portfolio as a collection of hard copy documents or computer files related to your working life. These different pieces of evidence or portfolio items can be arranged or rearranged to produce different versions of portfolio depending on the purpose. The different types and forms of evidence in a portfolio are organised specifically to meet the requirements of those who will read or assess the portfolio. The format of portfolios will also vary depending on the structure or use of a prescribed template such as an assignment requirement. These are usually recommended by educational course requirements or structured around records of employment or basic and continuing educa-tion. Compilations of hard copy documents are probably the most familiar portfolio format; however, developments in knowledge, information and learning technologies have prompted the emergence of digital or electronic portfolios as discussed in greater detail in Chapter 2.

As Figure 1.1 shows, professional portfolios commonly include résumés, education certificates, registration certificates, employment records, perfor-mance appraisals, references, letters and other related documents such as records of committee membership or volunteer activities. Personal reflective

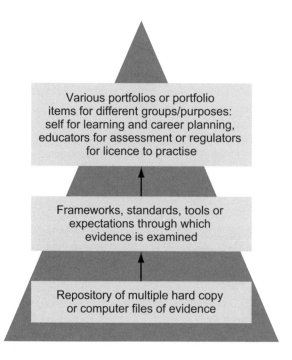

FIGURE 1.1 Portfolio components

statements trace the processes that have occurred in achieving changes in practice, learning, experience, knowledge and skills. These reflective and critical accounts of practice or learning enable you as the portfolio author to demonstrate deep learning about complex practice issues. Examples of these types of statements would be experiences and improvements in ethical understanding or clinical decision-making, which can be difficult to demonstrate in other ways. This type of evidence can assist the portfolio reader such as your lecturer or employer to assess shifts or developments in learning and levels of competence.

Portfolios will contain multiple documents including both official and personal papers, some of which may remain confidential to the author and not be shared with others. Disclosure and self-protection are addressed in more detail in Chapter 2. Suggested portfolio structures are examined in Chapter 2 also; however, an example of a specific structure would be where professional standards or competencies are used as headings, with evidence that demonstrates the levels of knowledge, skill and performance.

Summary points

- A professional portfolio is more than a log of events or a set of practice or learning-related documents.
- A professional portfolio is a broad and structured mix of different resources. These resources are collected or produced through a career-long process of continuous professional development and result in various portfolio items or products that can be used for different purposes.

Why do I need a portfolio?

Portfolios are widely used to reflect on learning and professional development needs as well as demonstrate performance outcomes. The very nature of keeping a portfolio and reflecting on personal achievements and learning needs is in itself a useful exercise. However, the various portfolio items can be put to varied uses. The most common reasons for nurses and midwives to create a professional portfolio are to meet the performance review requirements of an employer or to assist in meeting the registration audit requirements of a regulatory authority. Across a career a nurse or midwife might also use a portfolio to apply for credit or exemption in studies as part of recognition of prior learning at university or apply for overseas registration. Portfolios also provide a personal resource from which to evaluate and plan career choices.

The following discussion examines some of the issues that impact on the need for nurses and midwives to develop skills in communicating competence.

Healthcare, health workforce and scopes of practice

There are increasing demands for new and more health services. Aside from global crises in economics and climate, other factors shaping the provision of health services include the growth and ageing of the population, the changes to the burden of disease and shift to focus on health prevention and consumers and workforce expectations (National Health Workforce Taskforce 2009). Managing the international flows of health professionals with different languages, cultures and educational preparation is an aspect of the health workforce that needs attention to enable quality healthcare.

Nurses are an active part of the worldwide labour market described by Kingma (2006) as 'brain drain', 'brain gain' and 'brain circulation'. Nursing, and perhaps to a lesser degree midwifery, is also affected by the emergence of new healthcare roles. Examples of these include the shift of personal care and lifestyle support responsibilities from nurses to carers. Any gap in this shift is occupied by nurses taking on new practices and decision-making responsibilities.

The increase in new health conditions, technologies and expectations demands that nursing and midwifery practice adapt and extend its scopes of practice (Heartfield 2006, National Nursing and Nursing Education Taskforce 2005, p 38). For the individual registered nurse this may mean practice beyond the established contemporary or 'traditional' scope of practice to include new technology, increasingly autonomous roles, management of health consumers with chronic conditions, and through activities previously considered within the scope of other health professionals (Nursing Council of New Zealand 2010). Government health policy and employer-based initiatives may also drive shifts in nursing and midwifery scopes of practice such as seen in recent announcements of new and reallocated funding for a range of nursing initiatives in Australia in rural, mental health and primary care areas (Russell 2010).

These circumstances, coupled with the focus on quality healthcare and patient safety, mean health professionals are subject to increased scrutiny. This scrutiny or monitoring is not only from within employing organisations or by peers or colleagues, but also from external bodies such as government and media and from the consumers of healthcare themselves.

For individual nurses and midwives there are two levels of impact from this situation. First, nurses and midwives need to understand their professional obligation to demonstrate their competency for professional practice. Secondly, because not all competencies can be observed or measured, nurses and midwives need to develop the skills to reflect on and communicate their levels of competency. It is the second of these requirements that the professional portfolio is designed to meet.

Regulation of professional practice

In addition to being subject to public scrutiny, nurses and midwives are subject to various layers of regulation. Regulatory frameworks for the health professions are complex and take various forms. They set out the different requirements for practice through both legislative and non-legal processes.

In Australia, a new regulatory authority, the Australian Health Practitioner Regulation Authority (AHPRA) has been formed by an Act of Parliament. From 1 July 2010, this national agency became responsible for the registration and accreditation of ten health professions in Australia. Along with nurses and midwives, the initial list of nationally regulated health professionals includes chiropractors, dentists (with dental hygienists, dental prosthetists and dental therapists), medical practitioners, optometrists, osteopaths, pharmacists, physiotherapists, podiatrists and psychologists. In 2012 the following professions will join the national scheme: Aboriginal and Torres Strait Islander health practitioners, Chinese medicine practitioners, medical radiation practitioners and occupational therapists.

AHPRA is bound by the Health Practitioner National Law Act (2009) which provides the regulatory framework for health practitioners. It makes specific reference to registration, accreditation, complaints and conduct, health and performance, and privacy and information sharing. A separate National Board has been formed to protect the public and set the standards and policies that regulate each of the initial ten health professions (Australian Health Practitioner Regulation Agency). Each state and territory has now passed legislation that cancels the previous health professionals Acts (including the various Nurses and Midwives Acts) and enacted the new national law. The nursing and midwifery titles that are covered by the Health Practitioner National Law Act 2009 are nurse, registered nurse, nurse practitioner, enrolled nurse, midwife and midwife practitioner (Health Practitioner Regulation National Law Act 2009). A new feature of this Act is that a register has been developed of all students undertaking approved programmes of study for registration as health professionals.

The Nursing and Midwifery Board of Australia does not specify that nurses and midwives should keep a professional portfolio though they do require documentation of continuing professional development and specify certain features of this documentation (Nursing and Midwifery Board of Australia). Nurses and midwives need to identify learning priorities and keep records of verifiable continuing professional development activities including outcomes and the number of hours spent on each activity. These records need to demonstrate that the nurse or midwife has:

1. evaluated their practice against the relevant competency or professional practice standards to identify and prioritised their learning needs
2. developed a learning plan based on identified learning needs

3. participated in effective learning activities relevant to their learning needs
4. reflected on the value of the learning activities or the effect of participation on their practice.

Since 2003 health professionals in New Zealand have been governed by the New Zealand Health Practitioners Competence Assurance Act (Nursing Council of New Zealand 2005a). This Act requires health practitioners (including nurses and midwives) to demonstrate their competence to practise and their professional education in new skills and technologies. Nurses and midwives in New Zealand are regulated by separate councils — the Nursing Council of New Zealand and the Midwifery Council of New Zealand. The protected nursing and midwifery titles are registered nurse, midwife, enrolled nurse and nurse practitioner. In addition to the Australian nursing and midwifery titles, the Nursing Council of New Zealand regulates the nurse assistant role (Nursing Council of New Zealand 2005b). As in Australia students of nursing and midwifery undergraduate programmes are also listed on a register.

Understanding the regulation of nurses and midwives requires some understanding of competence. This may appear straightforward as nursing and midwifery regulatory authorities provide various codes, guidelines, standards and competency statements. However, competence is a generic term referring to someone's overall capacity while competency refers to specific capabilities, such as nursing or midwifery or communication or leadership. The literature is confusing with terms used interchangeably and varying either between a focus on specific tasks within a role or on a more holistic view of competence where the focus is on the complexity of skill acquisition and application (Australian Primary Health Care Research Institute).

Despite the lack of clarity of definitions in the literature, it is clear that the approaches to competency-based education fall into one of two broad categories. There are probably as many types of competence as there are types of intelligence. It is for this reason that useful discussion of competence needs to address both the context in which the knowledge, skill and capacity are put into action as well as the overall level of competency in any specific area.

Self-regulation

Professional regulation also requires nurses and midwives to be active participants. If we consider the regulation of nurses and midwives by statute or law as mandatory, then there is also a voluntary aspect that needs to be acknowledged. Voluntary regulation involves nurses and midwives accepting that they are required to practise as individuals but within agreed boundaries and according to agreed standards (Bryant 2005). This idea of self-regulation of the individual (as opposed to self-regulation of the profession by the profession) assumes that individuals participate in a range of self-regulatory activities. For this to occur individuals need an internal locus of control that enables them to be accountable for understanding themselves as well as the requirements of the profession and the contextual demands of practice. One example of a self-regulatory activity is assessment of existing levels of competency and identification of learning needs for continuing professional development.

Clearly it is important that all nurses and midwives access the necessary information from the relevant authority fully to understand their obligations under the law and in relation to the relevant registration standards, codes and guidelines. Completion of the activities at the end of this chapter will help you develop the skills to stay informed about this type of development.

Resources

Useful websites to understand better nursing and midwifery regulation include the following:

Australian Health Practitioner Regulation Agency
http://www.ahpra.gov.au/
Midwifery Council of New Zealand
http://www.midwiferycouncil.health.nz/
Nursing Council of New Zealand http://www.nursingcouncil.org.nz/
Nursing and Midwifery Board of Australia
http://www.nursingmidwiferyboard.gov.au/

Other forms of regulation of nursing and midwifery practice

In addition to the health practitioner Acts, there are a number of other laws in the Australian states and territories that specify responsibilities for nurses and midwives. Examples of these are laws concerning therapeutic or controlled substances, mental health, aged care, mandatory reporting, immunisation and weapons.

Processes other than laws that regulate the way nurses and midwives practise include various health industry standards and accreditation processes, such as those developed to guide health and social care in particular contexts (e.g. aged care). The provision of healthcare services at the organisational level is also governed (that is regulated) through numerous levels and mechanisms which may be linked to funding or accreditation to provide services. Professional organisations such as colleges and special interest groups also play a role in shaping the practice of individuals and the professions through various lobbying, policy, guideline and standards development activities.

Employing organisations regulate nurses and midwives through organisational standards and the various industrial awards and agreements that specify roles and employment conditions such as salary and leave entitlements. Another form of professional regulation is where there is agreement by the members of a profession, or a subgroup of a profession, about a particular matter. This may be on levels of proficiency, such as advanced practice, or the use of specialist titles such as critical care nurse, lactation consultant or diabetes educator (National Nursing Organisations 2006).

Continuing competency requires the use of a professional portfolio by nurses and midwives in the United Kingdom and in New Zealand (Midwifery Council of New Zealand 2008, Nursing Council of New Zealand 2008, Hull et al 2005).

Summary points

- It is useful to keep a portfolio because nursing and midwifery as professional groups and individual nurses and midwives have a range of mandatory and voluntary professional obligations within which they are required to maintain agreed standards of practice.
- Portfolios provide a useful means to track changes in practice and performance as healthcare becomes increasingly complex and open to scrutiny through governance and audits of standards of care.

Activity: Building your portfolio

Finding answers to the following questions will help you to understand the links between keeping a professional portfolio and evidence of healthcare knowledge and skill development.

1. Who authorises or regulates your ability to practise as a nurse, midwife or other healthcare practitioner?
2. Who assesses your learning and development either as a student or in your employment position?
3. What do these individuals or organisations require as evidence of your ability to do your job successfully or to demonstrate learning?
4. Do they specify a template or format in which this information needs to be presented (such as annual performance reviews)?
5. Do they provide guidelines about the types, volumes or forms of evidence they require?
   In answering these questions it will be useful to use the internet to search for the specific codes, standards or guidelines that are used to regulate your practice. It is a good idea to know who produces or endorses these standards and how they are used to regulate your practice. They will be discussed in greater detail in subsequent chapters.
6. As a further activity you might expand your information search strategies (e.g. internet, email or telephone) to compare the competency standards or statements of different regulating groups,

such as nursing (registered nurses — enrolled or division 1 and 2), midwifery, nurse practitioners and physiotherapy or pharmacy. While all nursing and midwifery regulatory authorities in Australia accept the same nursing and midwifery standards, they also produce standards about specific aspects of practice and regulation (e.g. the use of restraint, medication management or approval of education providers). Review the New Zealand nursing competencies standards and learn about how New Zealand shares the same domains of competency. It is necessary for all regulated health professionals to be aware of the standards endorsed by their regulating body.

Reflection and lifelong learning

Most of us accept that change is constant and that we must learn the skills necessary fully to engage with what work and life have to offer. The concept of adult learning suggests that one of the reasons for adults being motivated to learn is because they understand that learning is necessary to be able to perform their professional or work roles (Knowles 1984). There are also links between the social and personal dimensions of our lives that impact not only on our individual professional growth and development, but also on the remaking and changing of professional practice (Billett 2006). Technology plays a key part in all aspects of our professional and personal lives and lifelong learning is seen as necessary in order to *develop* new technology, to apply new technology and to re-train for the new jobs that are created by new technology (Commonwealth of Australia 2005). The role of technology is particularly relevant and evident in this book in references to e-portfolios.

Lifelong learning skills equip nurses and midwives to manage the significant responsibilities of their roles. Lifelong learning skills include being

- information literate, which means being able to locate, evaluate, manage and use information in a range of contexts
- an effective communicator, which means being competent in the required level of reading, writing, speaking and listening
- self-aware, which means being able to understand and make maximum benefit of personal strengths and accept personal limitations
- contextually aware, which means being able to identify and find ways to manage the social, political, cultural and environmental influences on practice.

Recognition of the value of individual learning, within both formal and non-formal learning environments, has been the basis of the competency-based practice movement. This is evident in nursing and midwifery in most developed countries and certainly, as discussed earlier in this chapter, in Australia and New Zealand. These competencies and standards are used widely to inform educational programmes, clinical assessment and performance reviews, as well as for their core function as the basis for licensing for practice. They implicitly and sometimes explicitly require life-long learning and reflection on practice as indicators of competency.

So if we accept learning as a continuous part of professional practice then it is important also to understand that learning is more than just thinking about and remembering new information. We move from superficial or surface knowledge to a deeper understanding through complex psychological, social and emotional learning processes. Reflective thinking is one example of these processes (Hull et al 2005). Reflection is an important process in portfolio development. It is the examination or exploration of experiences with the aim of generating new understandings and appreciation (Boud et al 1985).

Reflection has a long history in nursing, midwifery and other health profes-sional educational programmes (Welch & Dawson 2006, Clouder & Sellars 2004, MacKenzie 2004, Baptiste 2005, Ward & Gracey 2006). This is because it is seen as a way to bring together knowledge and theory with practice or clinical actions. Knowledge is often understood to be developed through rational, processes of understanding scientific and theoretical information. However, we know that other types of knowledge come from other sources and the challenge for practice-based knowledge comes from linking theory, personal interpretation, experience and culture (Egan & Testa 2010, p. 153).

Reflective processes are attributed with making more apparent or obvious the knowledge and learning that occurs in practice (Palmer et al 1994, MacKenzie 2004). Skills in reflection help to differentiate between the facts that we know and how we interpret them and then how we might use this knowledge and interpretation in practice (Hull et al 2005). The widespread acceptance of reflection supports its potential in bringing together critical thinking, analysis, synthesis and evaluation of learning from practice in order to generate new learning and knowledge about practice (Clouder & Sellars 2004).

Summary points

· Lifelong learning involves both informal and formal learning and requires self-motivation to participate in learning to do an existing job, develop new ways of doing a job or retrain for a new job. Recognition of the value of individual learning, within both formal and non-formal learning environments, has been the basis of the competency-based practice movement.

· Practice-based knowledge is developed by reflective thinking, that is thinking through and developing links between theory, personal interpretation and experience and culture. Having reflective thinking and analysis skills help nurses, midwives and other health professionals to counteract the complexity of the health system, where often there are no prescribed right or wrong answers.

Portfolios and career planning

While much of the previous discussion has been looking back over practice to develop a case about competency for current practice, portfolios also have a major function in looking forward and developing a career plan.

Career planning is not just about a series of jobs. It is a lifelong investment and, as with any investment, planning pays off (International Council of Nurses 2001). A career is about purposefully linking your mix of employment and education to produce the best possible life that you want to live. The traditional idea of a job being for life is being replaced by more dynamic forms of working, including the now well recognised view that people need to play a greater part in the construction and development of their own careers (Haines et al 2006).

For the majority of nurses and midwives who work in the employment of others, the relationship with their organisation is an important consideration. While the focus of this relationship is mostly about performance, the role of organisations in career development has also changed. Employment is only one of a range of ways in which organisations help to shape an individual's career. Some other ways are providing education, training and credentials, brokering or mediating between individuals, and providing, protecting, enhancing, regulating and, of course, funding career development opportunities and activities (Kanter 1989). For the individual it is important to consider the way in which organisation-specific opportunities relate to broader developments in the health workforce. In most instances these changes are associated with technological advances and changing population profiles. An example is the way in which the ageing population and the move towards support for self-management of chronic conditions are demanding new skill sets in the health workforce.

The following principles highlight that career planning is more than setting individual goals for hierarchical progression within organisations (Haines et al 2006):

- change is constant, requiring people to recognise and value their fluidity and develop resilience
- career development is a lifelong journey, requiring individuals actively to engage in learning throughout life
- individuals benefit from being empowered and confident proactively to design and manage their preferred future
- an array of personal, family, social and environmental factors shape the development of career competence
- careers prosper where people seek the support of others and provide support to others
- communities prosper where individuals are empowered to make informed life, learning and work decisions.

The notion of career pathways in Australian nursing has often been interpreted narrowly as meaning the development of nursing classifications that exist in industrial awards and agreements (Price et al 2001) or the view that nursing and midwifery were located only within organisations so career issues were only industrial ones. More recent research shows that nursing students often enter programmes with preconceived ideas about their careers and where they will work after they graduate (Hayes et al 2006). Without exposure to different areas of practice these ideas may not change.

Career planning for nurses and midwives now recognises how changes in healthcare have resulted in considerable changes for nursing and midwifery professions and, therefore, for individual nurses and midwives. These changes included new roles and responsibilities, with a greater requirement not to limit career planning to what organisations have to offer, but to consider employment and career options more broadly. Awareness of projected changes in healthcare, such as the impact of ageing populations and shifts towards interdisciplinary and more community-based healthcare, generate opportunities for health practitioners to take more active responsibility for their futures. An example might be to think more broadly about identifying the education programmes best suited to accommodate trends in health service delivery. The growth in public and population health programmes and quality improvement and risk management are examples of such trends relevant to health practitioners.

The impact of change is evident in the International Council of Nurses' recommendation that nurses become career-resilient by being flexible and adaptable (International Council of Nurses 2001). The following discussion examines how portfolios can assist in career planning.

Career planning steps

The process of planning and developing a career is an integral part of ongoing professional development. Self-awareness and self-observation are core skills for nurses' professional development (Donner & Wheeler 2004) Career development is a continuous iterative process of moving back and forth between the phases of work, life and learning whereby strengths and limitations, career visions and plans are evaluated (Donner & Wheeler 2004). Career planning allows you to capitalise on your motivation and make informed decisions (or overcome poor motivation or continued indecision) and focus your efforts towards purposefully set career goals.

As previously discussed, portfolios provide a way for you to review, refine, evaluate and re-evaluate both your current situation and your goals and progress plans for the future. Goal-setting is a process that can motivate people and therefore assist in achieving short- and long-term goals. Goals need to be linked by an overarching vision of what you want to achieve in your working life and the personality, values, beliefs, skills and work interests that are rewarding to you. It is important for nurses and midwives to set goals to ensure that they plan not only their future employment but also their career pathways; they need also to work out contingency plans in case their goals are not met. Understanding, predicting and attending to changing healthcare deliveries will further enhance the likelihood of meeting your personal goals.

Portfolios offer a place in which to store all the information relevant to your nursing or midwifery career. The portfolio development process outlined in this book involves self-reflection and evaluation of your knowledge, skills, current practice and experiences, as well as analysis of other perspectives, the available evidence and generated new evidence. This is followed by the development of statements that outline the evidence, skills and learning and a sound argument for development and achievement. In this way, portfolios help describe your professional strengths and limitations, and can be used as a marketing and self-promotional tool as well as submitted during the application process and referred to during job interviews. Portfolios also provide a career development plan that overrides daily work activities and pressures. It can focus what you do at work and help you to manage workplace stresses and demands and prepare yourself for change.

Portfolios provide a basis from which better to understand your preferences and skills in ways that show your suitability to certain nursing or midwifery contexts or areas of work. By looking for trends in performance evaluations or other forms of feedback, a professional portfolio can act as a map to the things that need to be done to progress your career decisions and plans. A portfolio may highlight areas that can be raised in performance review sessions for future development. To achieve this, portfolios need to be examined as an entire collection of experiences. This collection is then organised not only according to competencies but also to past achievements and strategic plans that address personal or organisational goals. In using a portfolio for career planning, the details need to be organised with attention to your strengths, limitations and preferences, as much as your achievements, experiences and expertise in areas of practice.

Career planning using a portfolio involves thinking beyond your current situation. Your aims are to think about what goals, roles or positions are to be achieved, what actions need to be taken and with what resources and, lastly, how you will know when you have reached or achieved your goals. Career planning requires self-assessment, research into your area of work, decision-making and goal-setting, regular reviews of résumés and periodic reviews of job opportunities.

Resources

The International Council of Nurses website includes career-planning information (International Council of Nurses 2001). This material provides sets of questions about your interests, environment, goals and plans for action as well as how to evaluate all this. This resource can help you identify and consider your personal preferences, as well as the views of others who are important to your life and work. The questions are designed to help you develop career goals and identify the actions necessary to achieve these goals.

There are many career counselling resources and services available through internet searches or events such as open days and seminars provided by universities or professional organisations. Most universities provide generic career planning resources and services for new applicants or graduates. These may be available online or as individual counselling for students. The websites of government employment and education departments and some regulatory authorities and professional organisations often include career-planning tools and information. National and international professional organisations and government health department websites are useful places to visit to keep track of developments in healthcare and associated employment opportunities. Reading employment pages on a regular basis will also provide you with insight into the types of positions that are available and the associated requirements, remuneration and benefits. You will probably note, for example, the increase in nursing positions in quality and risk management, aged and community care, and general practice.

It is a good idea to discuss your career plans with others to get new information or ideas worth considering. This may also highlight other ideas or perspectives you had not thought about. Mentors, colleagues, family, friends and supervisors can provide valuable professional guidance. Mentoring can take place through informal relationships with people you already know, or through professional networks, workplaces, conferences and professional interest groups. A mentor is someone who helps you in your professional planning over an extended period of time. A mentor is not the same as a preceptor or supervisor, who is focused on what you have to do in your job. There are many online resources about mentoring but, because mentoring is about interaction with others, a better source may be to find the nursing and midwifery organisations that have links to mentoring opportunities. Alternatively, just getting out and networking with members of your profession may assist you in meeting like-minded, willing, experienced and appropriate people to help you develop your potential.

Summary points

- People play a significant part in the construction and development of their own careers. However, career planning is more than setting individual goals.

· Reflection on individual professional practice and the broader healthcare contexts prompts the identification of current and future learning needs that can inform the ways forward for career planning and development.
· Developing a professional portfolio helps you learn a process for reviewing and re-evaluating your goals and plans for the future, as well as providing a place to manage this information.

Activity: Identifying existing portfolio information and evidence

Lastly make a list of the documents you already have that relate to either your nursing or midwifery studies, or to your employment in either of these roles. You might even go and find the documents and put them in one place or scan and keep as one file on your computer.

Conclusion

In bringing this chapter to a close, portfolios have been presented as part of professional practice which is linked to understanding the individual and collective obligations of regulated nursing and midwifery practice. Nurses and midwives enter their professional practice following successful completion of a university degree. This education is designed to equip them with the skills for continued learning and employers and regulatory authorities will require individual professionals to continue this learning after entry to practise to achieve a quality health service. This responsibility includes the need to keep sufficient quality evidence of practice and performance. The Nursing and Midwifery Board of Australia's requirement for continuing professional development illustrates how this ongoing learning is a lifelong responsibility for continuing competence in nursing and midwifery practice.

This chapter has focused on portfolios for professional practice while also recognising that portfolios have a place in assessment of learning as part of educational programmes, organisational performance reviews and individual career plans. The focus on key developments in the regulation of nurses and midwives has set the scene for understanding that a professional portfolio is more than a means of collecting and reflecting on evidence of learning or practice. It is a way to communicate, showcase and improve skilled health-care practice with the collective aim of improving the quality of the health system by growing the intellectual capital.

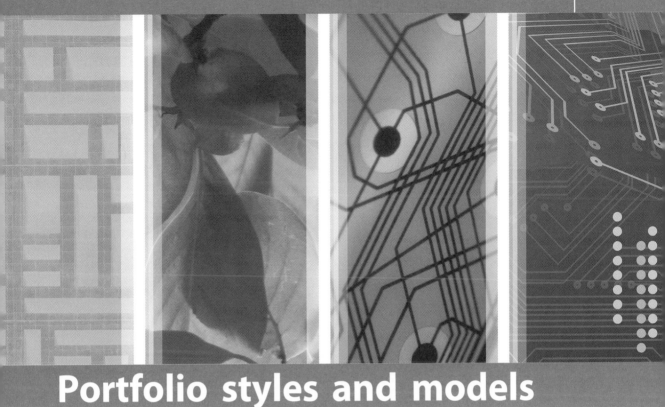

CHAPTER 2

Portfolio styles and models

Introduction

- Where do you start in designing your portfolio?
- What are the necessary and optional parts?
- What are the benefits and challenges of using an electronic platform to develop and display your portfolio?
- What are the challenges and potential risks in using electronic portfolios?

Moving on from understanding why it is necessary or useful to develop a professional portfolio, this chapter focuses on the variety of styles and models of portfolios as well as the purposes for which they might be used.

Searching the word 'portfolio' on the internet indicates the many uses of this term, as well as numerous formats, guides, templates and products. These are available from a variety of educational, commercial, regulatory and employment sources. Some guides are for purchase or are distributed as part of professional memberships, while others are available for free. Many of them are similar in design, with guidelines on how to bring together your career goals with your record of continuing professional development. This chapter will demonstrate how the main issue is not really which style you use

Nursing and Midwifery Portfolios. DOI: 10.1016/B978-0-7295-4078-0.10002-X

to develop a professional portfolio, rather, your format needs to support your intended portfolio use.

This chapter provides an overview of portfolio styles and features, followed by exercises for you to work through to help you meet the needs of your portfolio readership. The chapter ends with a detailed examination of electronic forms of portfolios or e-portfolios as the future of portfolio development.

What should my portfolio look like?

As mentioned in Chapter 1, most people start their 'portfolio journey' as a response to the expectations or requirements of an external group such as a university course, employer or regulatory authority. Alternatively you may put together a portfolio because you need evidence of job performance or because you are applying for a promotion or new job. The purpose of different portfolios will vary and it is important to think about your specific aim and other possible uses before choosing the design for your portfolio. Understanding the purpose of your first portfolio and through ongoing use you will come to value the suitability of some approaches over others. For example you may be a confident and regular computer user so the idea of an electronic portfolio is immediately appealing. Also your initial experiences in bringing together or creating relevant information (evidence) will introduce you to deciding how to tag or code them for possible future use.

Portfolio models

There are as many different formats of portfolios as there are purposes. Most nursing and midwifery portfolios are personal collections of employer or educator provided and self-constructed materials about education and practice, with some professional observations or reports on your practice by others. This chapter will extend this understanding of physical forms by introducing electronic or digital portfolios.

Before the move to electronic forms of portfolios, models were given names such as 'compilations', 'cake mixes' and 'toast racks' (Webb & Endacott 2002) in an attempt to illustrate how structured or unstructured portfolios might be, or their aims and outcomes. While all such models had their uses in career planning, educational assessment or performance evaluation, most had limitations. These included an overreliance on self-reported data and a lack of sufficient linking and explanation of evidence — what we refer to as development of an argument that demonstrates achievement. This also made portfolios very difficult to assess with any accuracy as reflected in the literature about assessing continuing competency (ANMC 2007, EdCaN 2008).

Figure 2.1 introduces a streamlined e-portfolio model. Portfolios are represented in this figure as having two interconnected spaces and functions; one

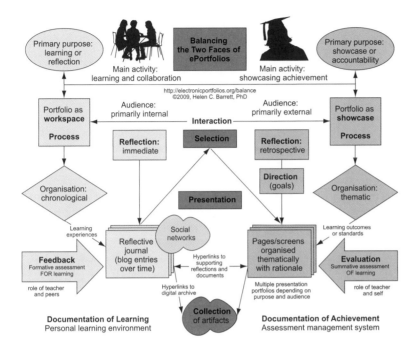

FIGURE 2.1 Portfolio dimensions (Barrett 2010)

is a workspace where learning and development occurs, and the other is a showcase where outcomes are demonstrated. Although the diagram refers to e-portfolios, the principles are also relevant to paper-based portfolios.

The workspace is process-focused in generating a repository of artefacts and personal information. Material is generated and stored chronologically with the main aim being to experience learning or reflection. The reflection is directed at a specific and recent experience or event (Barrett 2010).

The showcase is a product that displays accountability though arguments or stories that have multiple versions, be they public or private. These versions are available to varied audiences with access through varied permissions for a variety of purposes. The portfolio is for external audiences and is organised thematically around achievement, whether of standards, goals or learning outcomes. Reflection is about the past but directed at the future (Barrett 2010).

The components and interactions between these two portfolio 'faces' is explained further in the following chapters of this book.

What is an e-portfolio?

In its most basic form, an e-portfolio is a digital or computer-mediated space for storing materials, including text, images, video and sound, that can be drawn upon to produce one or more portfolios (AeP 2008). Initially e-portfolios were merely used to transfer text and images into electronic form, similar to that of an electronic curriculum vitae (Washington State University 2009). There are instances where there has been little progress beyond this, such that users compile their paper-based achievement records and convert these to electronic portable document format (PDF) files to enable them to submit via an online portal. This in itself is an advanced form of paper-based portfolios, as the original document remains with the individual, and depending on computer access, the submission process can be convenient and time efficient. This approach serves many institutions well, for having applicants submit documentary evidence in electronic form provides the convenience of not having to sort the post, file the various documents and maintain the paper records. However, as this chapter details, e-portfolios can also include additional supports to: assist with the development of artefacts; enhance reflective processes; extend learning and achievements via interaction with others; store and retrieve artefacts; and produce quality portfolio displays that depict the complexity of achievements through the inclusion of audio and visual images.

Who is the intended audience for my portfolio?

Although portfolios are likely to contain sections that are private and not designed to be read by others, most portfolios are written for an audience or specific readers. Knowing who your audience will be, and what their expectations are, is important in ensuring your portfolio is successful in communicating your intended message. In most cases the intended audience for a portfolio is external evaluators or assessors. Understanding the role of these people in reading and reviewing your portfolio is an important consideration when designing a quality professional portfolio. Consider whether there are criteria that will be used to evaluate your portfolio. If you plan to develop or use an existing portfolio in response to audit requirements by a regulatory authority, then they will evaluate your portfolio against the standards that outline your role and the safety of the public. They will know about the statutory requirements for nursing and midwifery and it is your responsibility to ensure they have the available best evidence to assess your knowledge, skills and practice. Therefore, there is little need for you to explain the regulations that inform and guide your practice, but rather you must demonstrate that you are aware of the range of regulations and give examples that illustrate your application of these in the clinical setting.

When applying for a job the most important information to obtain is the job description and selection criteria. Without these you may be offering knowledge and skills that do not match what the employer is seeking. A common frustration for selection or assessment panels is searching for the right information to appoint or pass an application. This frustration also occurs for panels when otherwise suitable applicants who do not address the required criteria are rejected for interview or appointment. Thus, it is in your best interests to show early in the portfolio the criteria that you will be addressing — hence the value of a product-orientated portfolio.

Using outcomes statements such as competency statements quickly directs the portfolio reader's attention to your preparedness to address the key criteria required. Once you have decided on the section headings, your main task will be to bring your evidence together and place it in the correct spots! In addition, you will of course need to develop a summarising statement justifying how your evidence meets the criteria. While this latter requirement may seem a little onerous, keep in mind that the structure/section headings are there to assist you.

How to collate your evidence and develop the narrative will be addressed in later chapters of this book. For now the focus will be on establishing the purpose of your portfolio, as well as developing an outline of a convincing argument about why your evidence of achievements meets your portfolio objectives.

What is the specific purpose of my portfolio?

The purpose of your portfolio is likely to be part of an educational assessment, position application, renewal of licence to practise, promotion application or application to a nursing or midwifery regulatory authority for professional status. As Figure 2.1 indicates, portfolios will have a repository section where you store and develop (process) portfolio items as well as the product aspect where you compile the portfolio version for the particular audience. In producing the portfolio product there will usually be some criteria to use as the structure for that version of your portfolio. Remember that the aim of a portfolio is to provide an audit trail of reasoning to support the arguments or claims of achievement made in your portfolio. Where there are set criteria it makes sense to use these as the headings and subheadings in your portfolio. For this reason it is imperative that you check whether such criteria exist and that you fully understand what they mean. The selection criteria that will guide you in designing your portfolio framework are generally available via the internet, an organisation's human resources department or an educational course coordinator. In some instances, further explanation is available through printed texts for purchase, for example the Nursing and Midwifery Board of Australia/ANMC competency cues and scope of practice decision-making frameworks provide useful detail (Nursing and Midwifery Board of Australia 2006). It is also worth noting that using a different set of criteria or headings to those specified may frustrate your portfolio readers when information is not readily accessible. If you are using a different framework or structure it is recommended that you cross-reference your framework with the specific criteria or information that was requested by those who will read the portfolio.

Where criteria do not exist or you are putting together a portfolio for your own career development purposes, you must decide on a suitable framework. While examples are provided in later chapters, a common framework for a nursing or midwifery portfolio would be to use the professional competency statements or other relevant regulatory guidelines.

Summary points

· Portfolios may be paper-based or in electronic form.
· They provide a repository space for the portfolio author to collect information and evidence and process and develop particular skills. They also enable the production of various forms of portfolios to be made available to different audiences.
· Portfolios communicate a message to the reader so it is important to understand and decide on the specific purpose of each version of your portfolio, including who will be reading and evaluating the portfolio.

Activity: Building your portfolio

If you have not done so previously make notes now about why you are thinking of developing a portfolio and for what purpose.

· What is the reason you are putting together a portfolio? Is your portfolio for your personal use? If so, is it for you to plan your career or attend to your personal learning goals?
· Are you planning to use your portfolio as evidence to seek or maintain registration?
· Is your portfolio part of an assignment for an educational programme? If so, what are the objectives or assessment criteria that will direct your portfolio construction? A common aim of assessments that require the development of a portfolio is showing you have the skills to develop evidence of your learning. Think about the sort of picture you plan to paint of yourself as student or practitioner.

Use a single sentence to explain the purpose of your portfolio. Then consider the following:

· What outcomes do you need to demonstrate — competency statements, performance standards, role specifications, etc?
· Who is your audience? Who will be evaluating this portfolio and what will they need to know?

Privacy, confidentiality and disclosure

Healthcare practitioners have important legal and ethical responsibilities with regard to privacy, confidentiality and disclosure. The fundamental principles of privacy include fair and lawful collection of information, choice and transparency in the use of data, accuracy in data quality, appropriate data security and access for individuals to their own information (Curtis 2005). Australia and New Zealand have specific national privacy legislation, as well as various amendments, state and territory legislation and industry codes and guidelines, resulting in complex regulation of privacy for both the government and private sectors (Office of the Australian Information Commissioner 2006).

For the health sector, the obligations of providers as specified in the privacy acts are expected to complement professional and ethical obligations regarding confidentiality contained in the various professional codes of ethics and conduct. Healthcare consumers are entitled to expect that all health practitioners will maintain a high standard of confidentiality — disclosing information to others only for the purposes of treatment (National Health and Medical Research Council 2004).

The implications of privacy laws when compiling a professional portfolio are that careful attention must be given to protecting the identities of anyone mentioned in the portfolio. This means modifying details about all patients, health practitioners or anyone else to whose information you have access through your employment or practice and which may be included in your portfolio. Names of persons need to be removed or changed. In some cases you may also need to change the details of an event or situation so that a person or persons cannot be identified. For example, if you include a case study or care plan in your portfolio, it is not only the name of the patient but also the names of the family, doctors and other health providers that need to be removed or changed. Where an individual is named in a portfolio, a statement should be made explaining that all identifying features have been removed or changed. Depending on the context of what is being written about, there may also be circumstances in which organisations need to be de-identified. However, if someone provides you with a signed document such as a reference or performance assessment, it is appropriate for this person's name and title to be detailed in your portfolio.

In compiling a portfolio the concept of confidentiality could be used as a tag or code to mark items of evidence. For example an evidence item might be tagged as open for disclosure to all portfolio audiences or restricted to personal reading.

Another consideration when compiling a portfolio is personal disclosure. We have suggested that you consider carefully the audience of your portfolio to ensure you send the right message to the readers. You also need to protect your own interests in the information you share. Any document you submit for professional reasons — either for assessment as part of a course or performance review, or re-licensing as a nurse or midwife — may be scrutinised by a number of people and in some cases may become the property of others. While your information should not be used for any additional purpose without your consent, it is useful to remember that there are processes such as subpoenas and freedom of information applications by which documents can be released to the public, the media or the courts. You are therefore advised to think carefully about the written disclosure of personal reflections, opinions about events or people, and personal diaries used to record work-related matters.

Organisation and presentation of portfolios

Previously portfolios were most often associated with bulky binder folders and plastic sleeves. Certainly the developing and evolving nature of portfolios necessitates the movement of information and, as previously discussed, the use of computers and development of e-portfolios has changed this process considerably. We would therefore recommend to anyone starting out that you consider developing your portfolio in the format of electronic files. This will require a little extra work initially in getting or developing a template and learning how to scan the necessary documents (e.g. hand-written appraisals). The initial inconvenience will, however, become insignificant when you come to storing, assembling and distributing your portfolio in electronic form (e.g. on a CD-ROM).

Whether you compile your information electronically or in a binder folder, a neat professional product is the objective. A title page, table of contents, clear sections and so forth are standard requirements. The example of a portfolio structure in Table 2.1 may be useful to consider.

The objective of Table 2.1 is to build on Figure 2.1 and provide you with a visual sense of what might be included in a portfolio. As you can see, a portfolio has the potential to be a substantial document. However, do not be fooled into thinking that volume equates to quality: quite the contrary — a voluminous portfolio filled with certificates may communicate an inability to evaluate and discern relevance and worth. The aim is to provide *concise* evidence that you are competent to practise in your particular role, or the one you are aiming to work in, so the focus needs to be on the relevant competencies or standards, with the evidence and argument for how you meet them. As will be illustrated in the following chapters, the quality of the various portfolio entries is important in communicating an understanding of quality practice.

In moving on to consider what a portfolio might look like it is useful to understand about electronic or e-portfolios and how these might differ from paper-based approaches.

TABLE 2.1 Example portfolio structure

1. Table of contents
2. Portfolio explanation — details of the purpose and use of the portfolio
3. Personal details — this may be extended into personal profiles/curriculum vitae
4. Placement-experience record/work-experience summary
5. Competency statements or standards (not listed and dependent on portfolio purpose)
6. Appendices such as
   · learning objectives and associated achievements
   · employment summaries
   · role descriptions
   · professional practice assessment forms
   · completed case studies, concept maps and other related assignments
   · a reflective journal
   · medication calculation assessments
   · certificates of attainment (e.g. manual handling, cardiopulmonary resuscitation)
   · completed clinical skills assessment checklists
   · summaries of activities/tasks undertaken
   · academic transcripts
   · referee reports and testimonials
   · care plans and other work-related documents

E-portfolios

We now move on to extend the introduction to e-portfolios, particularly as represented by Barrett (2010). The focus is examining the differences in using the electronic medium to produce and manage portfolios for learning and/or showcasing achievements. A key feature that will be discussed is the role of reflection in shaping portfolios regardless of the portfolio medium. It would be a mistake to assume that by using an electronic portfolio (e-portfolio), the technology will remove or reduce the need to reflect on your practice or learning. If you find yourself merely following a menu and uploading files without considering the connections between your achievements, your learning and your future goals then you need to ask yourself, 'is this really a portfolio activity'? This warning is not intended to put you off e-portfolios, rather to highlight that there is the potential for some institutions/organisations to misuse the term e-portfolio to include the uploading of files with no inherent reflective process. It is important to note that using the electronic medium to store, structure and present portfolios does provide different opportunities and challenges from paper-based approaches. In addition to including digital/electronically mediated files such as video clips, blog entries and online learning tools, e-portfolio platforms also include search facilities to manage files, plus templates to structure and present your work. Learner-centred individualised learning, lifelong learning, reflection and peer learning are central to e-portfolio developments (Joyes et al 2010).

With the advent of the e-learning and associated e-portfolio industries, e-portfolios are becoming commonplace in education programmes and institutional regulatory processes. Hence, it is important that you understand the benefits and pitfalls of e-portfolios to enable you to reflect critically on the value and application of this burgeoning field.

The emergence of e-learning and the associated technologies to support personalised online learning has reignited the enthusiasm for portfolio learning and in effect initiated the e-portfolio industry. In part, it is because of this emerging e-portfolio industry that there can be confusion about the term 'e-portfolio'. The term e-portfolio has been used to describe: the software; a single portfolio submission undertaken in electronic form; or, all items/artefacts within a portfolio repository (Stefani et al 2007). Within the context of this book, the term e-portfolio will be used to describe the various components of a portfolio activity undertaken electronically. More specific terms such as 'e-portfolio platform' will be used to describe the associated software programs marketed to support portfolio activities online. The term 'e-tools' will be used for the learning and other professional activities that can be used to develop and record portfolio artefacts via the online medium. The portfolio displayed online in a web page format, with imbedded web links and other electronically mediated information, will be referred to as a web-folio.

Figure 2.2. illustrates the potential components of an e-portfolio.

As the figure shows, an e-portfolio software program/platform may include an array of components. There are a range of specific e-portfolio software

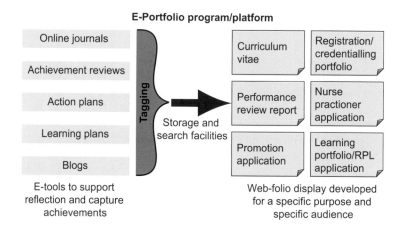

FIGURE 2.2 Schematic representation of e-portfolio components (Andre 2010, p. 121)

programs available such as Mahara, PebblePad, Desire2Learn, FolioTech or Chalk & Wire. These computer programs are designed to support the electronic construction, storage and display of the various portfolio components. In most instances, individuals are able to access these programs for a fee or as part of Open Source software program arrangements. Each program has different emphasis and may or may not include the specific components displayed in Figure 2.2.

E-portfolio programs also provide a convenient space/repository to save your work in a space-efficient form. Depending on the program, this information can be stored locally such as on a personal computer and data stick, or remotely via a server site that can be accessed at different locations online. The remote access is particularly useful when sending others a link to your web-folio, as there are no issues with file size or software requirements (Stefani et al 2007).

It is possible for a 'computer savvy' individual to put together an e-portfolio without using a specific e-portfolio program. For instance, there are numerous personal web pages used by individuals to display and develop their learning and achievements that are quite separate from a formal e-portfolio software program. Many of these integrate online blogging, journaling or related activities to reflect upon and extend their skills. As many educational institutions have identified, however, formal platforms provide useful supports and structure for students to develop their skills and understandings associated with portfolio activities. In effect, e-portfolio platforms can become personal learning spaces, where individuals can develop their learning independently from formal educational input, store artefacts developed in educational and professional environments and then use these to plan and design future learning opportunities.

It is not the purpose of this text to provide recommendations for e-portfolio platforms. However, by understanding the general functions of e-portfolios, you will be in a good position to decide upon a program that addresses your needs. Each of the groups of components depicted in Figure 2.2 will be addressed individually in the following materials.

What are e-tools?

An important facility of most e-portfolio platforms is the ability of students/ users to invite others to view and comment on their e-tool products, other artefacts or web-folio pages. The convenience of doing this online, plus the security of invitation processes, is an important feature of the e-learning experience. In most instances, artefacts can be shared and developed online in collaboration with peers, and submitted to staff for formative assessment. Some e-tools, such as wikis and blogs, include facilities to generate reports about the contributions of group members, which can be used as part of the assessment and conflict resolution processes.

Through the combined development of the e-learning and social networking industries, there is now an array of e-tools suitable for e-portfolio activities. Which e-tools you might need, if any, is clearly a personal decision. Increasingly there are some important blog and wiki sites where professionals can exchange ideas and support group learning. For many professionals, these 'communities of practice' provide an important resource to support and extend their learning through bench-marking and exchanging ideas and resources (Evans & Powell 2007). Students exposed to class discussion boards will be familiar with this approach, whereby individuals can upload documents and other resources for their colleagues to comment on. As with class discussion boards, professional blogs and wikis may have restricted access to allow only those invited to contribute to access the site. Setting up a blog or wiki is quite simple; the costs vary according to the size of the site and the level of access restriction. Hence, setting up a 'community of practice' for a group of clinical specialists can be readily achievable. Importantly, for a community to be successful, you need to have shared interests and goals, with members having a genuine interest in achieving a shared outcome (Santy & Smith 2007). A link to a wiki or blog site in your portfolio can then be a demonstration of your leadership, critical thinking and analysis, collaborative practice or any number of professional competencies. As will be elaborated upon later in this chapter, transferring e-portfolios to paper will mean that the quality of these sorts of activities will be lost. The interactive and collaborative nature of a blog or wiki site provides a level of professional authenticity that cannot be easily demonstrated in a paper-based artefact. A web link is meaningless unless accessed, and so if converting your portfolio to a paper form you may need to include excerpts from the site as an appendix. While not totally satisfactory, this would still be a very useful artefact.

Although not completely necessary, you can also use an e-journal to record and reflect upon your thoughts and extended readings.

Resources

There are several journaling software programs available, for example LifeJournal (http://www.lifejournal.com/), The Journal (http://www. davidrm.com/thejournal/) and iPhone/iPad applications.

In addition to the facility to write quickly and legibly, these applications/ programs can include functions such as voice recording and voice recognition software, tagging and search facilities to recall materials and prompts to encourage deeper reflection. Any note-taking system can also be used to record thoughts and reflections. These become particularly useful when associated with e-books and e-libraries, where you can search and tag information from multiple sources, imbed references and structure your own reflective journal. Links to these facilities, or excerpts from these journals, can be stored within your e-portfolio repository and inserted within a specific portfolio/web-folio as a demonstration of your reflective skills applied to practice.

For those of you familiar with the use of concept maps to cluster and conceptualise information, programs such as Mindjet/MindManager are useful, and can be accessed by others if converted to a Word document. If, however, you do not use concept maps often enough to justify the cost of purchasing a specific software program, photographing the map you have drawn on your white board, or converting your hand-drawn paper versions to a PDF, can be equally useful. A PowerPoint slide, Word document or program such as Prezi (http://prezi.com/) are other alternatives. Constructing a concept map can be useful in reflecting on and structuring complex tasks. The map also provides an important artefact that demonstrates your thinking in a succinct 'snap shot'.

All of the e-tools listed here have the potential to support the user in undertaking reflective activities and produce artefacts that illustrate a depth and complexity of professional practice. As previously mentioned, it is not necessary to use e-tools to achieve this; however, the benefits of the collegial exchange, ease of use and authentication aspects may well tempt you to consider using one or more of these in your repertoire.

What is tagging?

One of the advantages of an e-portfolio platform is that it provides a repository for the user to save and store digital artefacts. Documents such as learning plans, performance review reports, care plans and presentations can be saved directly as Word documents or as PDFs. Video clips, photos, pod casts and blogs can also be saved within the site. Over time there can be quite an accumulation of artefacts and it can be difficult to remember the relevance of each. The facility to tag each item and then search according to these tags is therefore very useful. The facility to store and draw upon artefacts you have collected over time is useful in reflecting on past learning or achievement in order better to understand and map future learning and development.

Tagging is pretty much the same principle as coding in research. It is a form of analysis which, at one level, aims to help overcome the challenges inherent in compiling potentially large volumes of information which can come from different sources and often in different forms. At another level, tagging or coding is putting into action a series of strategic decisions or allocating particular meaning to items of evidence. For example, this may be about how evidence items are different from or relate to each other and the portfolio aims. Coding or tagging is a way of managing information, partic- ularly when at the start it is difficult to know what pieces of information are most useful and what is destined for the rubbish bin. Tagging shows your logic or thinking and development of a style of portfolio development. It will often only be visible to the portfolio developer, with the portfolio audience only seeing the outcome but it is an important skill to develop and will be refined over the period of working on your portfolio. So this is why some clear thinking about the purpose of your portfolio and an understanding of models (such as process and product) will help manage your evidence at the early (as well as later) stages of portfolio development. The activities at the end of the chapter will direct you in creating your portfolio and the implications of this for an e-portfolio.

The e-portfolio platform allows the user to attach multiple tags for a single artefact. For example, you could tag an artefact according to the year produced and any number of professional competencies or role description headings. The aim is to capture whatever the artefact demonstrates as well as start to include issues you want to address such as the previously mentioned issue of confidentiality. The aim is to enable the portfolio producer, or maybe, with permission, the portfolio audience, to undertake a search according to specific tags or codes.

The benefit of multiple tags for a single artefact is a real plus when using an e-portfolio. As you have probably already identified, some artefacts can address any number of competencies or role descriptors. A case study, for example, can be a demonstration of understanding scope of practice, utilisation of evidence-based practice and quality communication skills. As has been discussed earlier, it is quite appropriate to use the same artefact as evidence for several categories in your portfolio, as long as the relevance to each category is apparent in the explanation.

It is very useful to consider your 'tag' categories early when developing your portfolio catalogue. It is useful to consider the likely purpose of future portfolios, for example for accreditation, position and promotion applications and performance review documents are likely. Given this, the categories associated with each of these are a likely source of tag categories. Examples of this would be:

· ANMC domains
· performance review categories
· the year the artefact was produced
· common position/promotion selection criteria.

As previously identified, an e-portfolio platform can provide a useful repository to store items in a space-efficient form, either locally, such as on a personal computer and data stick, or remotely, via a server site that can be readily accessed at different locations. In some respects this 'repository' is a computer-based filing cabinet. The tagging and search facility is a useful way of keeping track of the various items, and accessing them quickly and conveniently when developing a new portfolio for a specific audience.

Display function — for a specific purpose and specific audience

As has already been emphasised, when producing a portfolio to display to an audience it is particularly important to consider the purpose of the portfolio. As we progress through our careers we will need to produce different port-folios for different reasons. A promotion application is quite different from an application for recognition for prior learning, for example. An e-portfolio platform is useful in the construction of different portfolios for different purposes. Most platforms also provide a secure site to invite an audience to view your work. The following section will provide an overview of what a web-folio is and the benefits of using this approach. As has been previously identified, however, many institutions have yet to engage fully with digital and computer technology and so currently require paper-based portfolio submissions. As previously noted this will reduce some of the benefits of using hyperlinks to live reputable sites; however, with a little work you will be able to produce a credible portfolio document that draws on an array of artefacts to substantiate the claims made.

A web-folio is a portfolio displayed as a website, with a combination of headings, text explanations and embedded digital artefacts to provide evidence to support the claims being made. There are any number of websites available, not necessarily web-folios, that readily show the components and possible appearance of a web-folio. A quick online search can help understand how a web-folio might look, including the possible variations. Most web pages also contain text explanations that provide the context and meaning of the content. Hyperlinks and pictures within the text provide ready access to evidence and related sites. Designing your own web-folio/website format is not overly difficult, particularly if using an e-portfolio platform that includes facilities to assist.

Most website development and e-portfolio programs provide facilities to structure your page and limit site access to invited guests. In addition to providing valuable security and design assistance, having your artefacts stored within these sites reduces the problems of file size and audience access. It is, however, important to save your artefacts using software that is readily accessible to others. For instance PDF and Adobe software are commonly used for this purpose.

As with any portfolio, the structure and content of a web-folio needs to support the portfolio purpose, such that the audience are able to grasp the relevant information quickly. Headings that address the essential criteria, for example, are a useful structural approach. It is important that explanations are provided about the claims being made and relevance of the specific artefacts used to substantiate these claims. Unlike a paper-based portfolio, there is no need for appendices, rather the artefacts are inserted either directly (e.g. photos within the text) or as hyperlinks that then take the reader to the specific artefact. These allow the reviewer readily to access and evaluate the artefacts as they move through your presentation.

Some institutions, universities and other educational institutions in particular, have developed templates to assist e-portfolio users to develop their web-folios. In addition to enhancing the professionalism of the production, these templates may also assist the user to structure their portfolio and argument to suit the intended purpose. Hence, institutions are likely to develop several templates, each one addressing a different portfolio purpose. There is potential for these institutionally generated templates to include pre-populated information such as individuals' details, university grades and clinical reports. Those of you who have had to cut and paste information laboriously between performance review documents would no doubt appreciate the convenience of having some of this background information preloaded. This facility does not only support consistency in portfolio formats, but also, by having the background information preloaded, students and employees can focus on the reflective tasks of planning and framing their argument.

The artefact repository and search function is clearly a useful facility in producing the various web-folios/portfolios. As previously mentioned, no matter the format, an argument about the learning attained or performance demonstrated needs to be made in order for a portfolio to achieve its purpose. Reviewing all the artefacts within a specific category is a useful point to contemplate the argument that might be used. From a learning perspective, it is useful to revise artefacts that you produced early in your development, and reflect on the learning that has since been achieved. Similarly, the argument of competence can be framed as a progressive and culminating achievement. In doing so, you are communicating the application of generic skills such as a commitment and ability to develop as a professional. Hence reflecting on the scope, quality and progression of the artefacts you have collected is a useful exercise when considering the text that will support the various items of evidence within your portfolio.

The need to develop a paper-based or Microsoft Word document portfolio from an e-portfolio repository or web-folio is disappointing as some of the value and accessibility of the digital data is lost. However, it is an achievable and unfortunately sometimes necessary activity to develop a portfolio in print form. In situations such as this, using an e-portfolio platform to develop, store and retrieve artefacts is still a valuable exercise. As previously explained, e-tools can provide useful supports in producing structured and reflective artefacts, though unfortunately audio and video artefacts provide a particular challenge if you are required to make a document-based portfolio submission. The storage and retrieval capacities of an e-portfolio platform are also a very convenient way of managing and accessing your information. All of these facilities can still be useful in developing your paper-based portfolio. The real difference is that rather than imbedding your artefacts as hyperlinks within your portfolio text, you will need to include these as appendices.

Depending on the institutional requirements, it may not be possible to submit sound and video footage; however, printed versions of blog sites, e-journal entries, documents and PowerPoint slides are all achievable. At times it may be appropriate to include hyperlink addresses, particularly if this is an external source that provides verification of your achievement such as an online journal article or conference presentation. As previously noted, while it is disappointing that there are times when a web-folio cannot be used, it is possible to take advantage of the convenience of an e-portfolio platform and yet produce a documents-based portfolio submission.

Issues with/limitations of e-portfolios

Yes e-portfolios have their limitations. If you were hoping that this technology was somehow going to produce a well structured reflective portfolio after a few button clicks, then alas you will be disappointed. While e-portfolio platforms provide a convenient way to develop, store and retrieve artefacts and structure web-folios, it can be a mistake to associate this with simplifying the cognitive and reflective practices in developing and maintaining a portfolio. Ideally, as students are introduced to portfolios within their programmes of study, they will be supported progressively and incrementally to develop the skills and understandings associated with portfolio learning and development. However, while this support may assist these students, they too will be required to undertake contemplative and reflective exercises in producing their portfolio products. The real value of using portfolio is the individualized and applied learning/profession extension that is achieved as part of the process. Unfortunately technology has not, as yet, replaced the work needed to achieve this.

As many educational institutions have recognised in setting up e-portfolio platforms, ease of use and reliability of the technology is an absolute prerequisite. Complicated processes, non-intuitive instructions and failures in the technology, while increasingly less of an issue, are all potential risks when using an e-portfolio platform. If you are intending to use an e-portfolio platform, it is important to select a platform that meets your specific needs, abilities and resources. Most platforms are relatively reliable; however, problems do occur when working on underpowered computers or accessing online information via inadequate bandwidths. If you are trialling a product, it is recommended that you try uploading a range of files from the computer you intend to use. Also, be prepared to spend some time in learning the requirements of the program. Most programs come with instructional text and videos; four or five sessions of 30 minutes each should be adequate to be able to undertake most activities.

Moving between platforms can also be irritating and time consuming. For this reason, most educational institutions provide students with e-portfolio access after graduation, sometimes at a small fee. However, it is possible in most instances to transfer files to another platform if need be. Unfortunately, this can be time consuming and cumbersome, so you might want to consider this when deciding on a platform.

Social networking and other online environments have the potential for misuse and, as in any environment, bullying, misuse of others work, breaches of confidentiality and other forms of professional misconduct are all potential problems. However, possibly as a consequence of a misplaced sense of anonymity, ease of access or lack of understanding, breaches of netiquette (online etiquette) are unfortunately a problem. Breaches of confidentiality and other forms of unprofessional conduct, while possible in any situation, are easily exploited and communicated to others in the online environment, and so it is important to consider your own professional conduct online and protect yourself from the misconduct of others.

When circulating your portfolio artefacts or web-folios online try to use PDF documents rather than Word files that can more easily be copied, used and altered. While not a complete deterrent to the knowledgeable individual who can convert PDF materials into standard text, this would be a breach of professional protocol. Also be particularly careful about the standard of your work, do not use the work of others uncited, and ensure that the confidentiality of your clients, colleagues and institution is maintained.

It is important that your audience is also aware of their responsibilities about netiquette, providing quality feedback and not misusing other people's materials. Most institutions have policies about misuse of intellectual property and so if you are working in a professional environment you should have a level of protection. Unfortunately, theft of others' work does occur in all environments and the accessibility of materials in the online environment makes this a particular problem. Most institutions will insert disclaimers about this within the e-portfolio templates. The codes of conduct that guide our professional practice are also relevant in the online environment (Santy & Smith 2007). Issues of confidentiality, professional accountability to maintain standards of practice and ethical requirements to protect others apply in all professional settings. In addition to understanding this for yourself, if developing your own blogs or other professional exchange environments, it would be useful to consider including a policy statement drawing others' attention to this. It is important to highlight the professional purpose of such a site and reinforce the standard professional responsibilities of only using a resource for its intended purpose, ensuring that submission and responses maintain the rights of all individuals and the responsibility of others in monitoring and managing these standards. While the people with administrative responsibilities for blogs or other social networking sites have specific responsibilities to act when a breach of professional conduct occurs on their own site, we all have a professional responsibility not to sanction misconduct.

If not managed well, assembling e-portfolio artefacts and web-folios can be time consuming and irrelevant activities. It can be tempting for those who enjoy computer-based activities to spend considerable time compiling numerous irrelevant and poorly structured artefacts in the mistaken belief that quantity equates with quality. It is important to remember that a portfolio need not include every possible item; rather it should be a sample of your best and most relevant work. While it is important to engage with new technologies, it is equally important not to be a victim of e-gimmickry. It is disappointing to read a portfolio that is full of 'bling and ping' but short on content and process. As Stefani et al (2007) identify, e-portfolios are only effective if students/users take responsibility for their learning.

So where are e-learning and e-portfolios heading?

Increasingly e-portfolios and e-learning are becoming standard practice within educational programmes. E-learning, where course materials and the associated communications are provided via a range of online media, is now widely used in most undergraduate and postgraduate education programmes. The benefits of this not only include enhanced access to those with suitable computing systems, but if designed well provide a more interactive and realistic form of learning than traditional paper-based correspondence learning. The use of videos, interactive virtual technologies and social media are the sorts of technological enhancements that underpin quality online educational programmes. These same technologies also provide the opportunity to enhance the support and delivery of health care to those outside of centres of excellence. For instance, telemedicine, the use of Skype and online meetings has enable greater access to experts and expert advice.

In addition to providing quality and accessible learning, students are increasingly able to use these technologies to evidence their learning outcomes. Videos of an individual's participation in a simulation activity, or pod casts of the staff development presentations, provide a level of detail and authentication that past educational practices could not. Further from this, feedback via online virtual communities demonstrating an applied understanding of problem solving, disaster planning and inter-professional practice for instance, can now be evidenced via e-technologies. The inclusion of personal reflections and feedback from experts in the field further enhance the impact of e-portfolio artefacts. Mobile learning technologies via mobile phones and electronic note pads and such like, are useful and accessible resources for recording learning activities and providing internet access in a range of settings. Uploading these to your e-portfolio and seeking feedback from your peers and others is increasingly becoming an option for most of us.

Summary points

Benefits of e-portfolios include the use of:

· Artefacts such as audiovisual displays and blog activities, that provide more comprehensive and authentic depiction performance outcomes.
· Enhanced reflection through the use of peer feedback and the inclusion of communities of practice.
· Accessible storage and retrieval mechanisms such that materials and e-portfolios can be assembled and accessed online.

Challenges and potential risks of e-portfolios include:

· The need to be access electronically to be truly meaningful.
· The potential to be distracted by the technology such that the exercise can be time consuming.

Activity: E-portfolios

To learn more about e-portfolios, search the term online. If you are enrolled in a university course or programme, open the university homepage and enter the word 'e-portfolios'. Most universities now offer some version of the e-portfolio for their students. Sometimes it is linked at programme or course level while at other times resources are available through career development services. If you are not a student search for e-portfolio information and examples through reputable search engines and follow the links. Follow the links to e-journals provided earlier in this chapter or look for examples of e-portfolios that vary from simple electronic Word files to interactive multimedia portfolios. Many are available free.

Steps and responsibilities in portfolio development and use

Table 2.2 offers a series of steps to take when developing a portfolio. They would be the same whether the portfolio was electronic or web-based, or presented as a hard copy. The table also suggests how responsibility for portfolio development and use might be shared between those who prescribe, require and evaluate the portfolio and those who develop the portfolio.

Two examples of different types of portfolios are presented in Tables 2.3 and 2.4. In the first example, a portfolio is developed as part of an application for

TABLE 2.2 Steps and responsibilities in portfolio development

Stage	What is required?	Who is responsible?
Identification	Identify current practice or prior learning. This should include knowledge, skills, values and attitudes	Portfolio developer
Comprehension and application	Describe how the knowledge, skills and values fit with the required standard. This standard may be in the form of course or learning objectives, professional standards or a relevant role or position description	Portfolio developer
Analysis and synthesis	Document (or post online in an e-portfolio) the information necessary to communicate how the different examples of learning and practice come together into a claim or series of claims of achievement. These claims would be grounded in, and supported by, evidence	Portfolio developer with assistance from guidelines or advice from the course, employment or regulatory authority staff
Evaluation	Determine the extent of learning or achievement in relation to standards or objectives. Decide whether this is a necessary or acceptable standard	Portfolio developer (before submission or posting); course, employment or regulatory authority staff (after submission or posting)
Recognition	Recognise and register achievement such as a pass mark, employment, or registration or certification for practice	Organisation

a job promotion. In the second example, a portfolio is developed as part of an application to a nursing and midwifery authority for nurse practitioner status. It is recommended that you spend some time considering both of these because by examining a range of portfolios you will come to understand the specifics of your own portfolio needs.

The aim of this chapter was for you to consider the format that might best suit your portfolio purpose. The array of portfolio literature and formats available are potentially confusing. Some clarity has been given through classifying approaches into some models with selection linked to portfolio purpose.

The chapter has also examined the increasing use of online and computer technologies. We are early in the expansion of online health delivery facilities such as telemedicine and online patient support programmes. E-learning is also becoming an important part of the health professional repertoire. Increasingly student and professionals are able to access online course materials, engage with communities of practice from both within and outside our areas of employment and develop personalised learning outcomes that reflect the context of our own professional practice and career

TABLE 2.3 Portfolio to accompany a promotion application

What is the specific purpose of this portfolio — including implications?	The objective of this portfolio is to support an application for job promotion. Therefore, the promotion criteria and job description are important elements to consider in the portfolio design — you need to decide which of these to use as your framework or whether to use and perhaps combine both. Having read carefully the application statement or requirements and spoken to the Chair of the selection committee, you may decide to use the promotion criteria as a framework but to use **_bold italics_** whenever addressing components of the new job description. You could also make reference to the overlap between these two criteria, because this indicates insight into the position and promotion requirements.
Who will be reading it — including implications?	In a promotion application it is likely to be the selection or promotion committee members who will read the application and portfolio. They can be assumed to be familiar with the details and requirements of the employing organisation — hence there may be no need for explanation of the promotion criteria. Where there is representation from other departments or, in some cases, other organisations or disciplines, they may not be as familiar with the professional regulatory requirements specific to this position. In this case it may be best to clarify your understanding of these requirements in a sentence or two.

plan. As a consequence, the benefit of digital technologies within a professional portfolio to support learning and better illustrate the breadth and depth of professional achievements is becoming a reality. It is important to note, however, an e-portfolio platform is not just about storing and retrieving digital artefacts; in many respects it can become your own personal learning environment, where you can manage and develop your learning online.

E-learning and e-portfolios cannot replace all aspects of learning and skill development; however, they do provide a useful adjunct to traditional learning methods. By utilising the benefits of digital artefacts, peer and self-evaluation, plus the storage and retrieval capacities of e-portfolios, the possibilities for students to undertake individualised learning is enhanced. The use of web-folios that demonstrate overall performance or learning provide important capstone learning opportunities, where students are able to understand the relevance of the components of a programme of study. This is similar to the experience of compiling a promotion application, for example, where through the process the applicant comes to understand how the various achievements have the potential to be built into a larger picture of their competence.

TABLE 2.4 Portfolio in application for nurse practitioner status

What is the specific purpose of this portfolio — implications?	The objective of this type of portfolio is to support an application for a designated role that carries a particular and high-level status — nurse practitioner. The nursing and midwifery regulatory authorities' nurse practitioner standards and any specified guidelines will need to be obvious as section headings in the portfolio. In the case of the *National Competency Standards for the Nurse Practitioner* (Australian Nursing and Midwifery Council) and *Competencies for Nurse Practitioners* (Nursing Council of New Zealand 2008), you might clarify your understanding of Standards 1 and 2 to avoid missing aspects of the requirements for this role.
Who will be reading it — including implications?	Panel members will have been nominated by the relevant regulatory authority committee appointed to review such applications. What are their fields of expertise? Do you think they are familiar with your specialty area? Might they have been nominated to the committee because of their educational and regulatory experience? Answers to all these questions will shape the information you need to provide and the format of the portfolio.

Activity: Portfolio models and structure

We recommend you work through the following activities because they are a continuation of the learning in this chapter and have been designed to help you build your portfolio. Chapters 3–6 will help you consider the content of your portfolio, including the concepts of quality of evidence.

· Look at the information you have already generated. How is this stored and organised? Are your items stored chronologically with evidence of reflection and leaning directed at a specific and recent experience or event?
· Is this information ready for sharing with others with evidence of practice competency or learning achievements evident?
· Which external audiences would require access to your portfolio and what information from them do you need before you can prepare your portfolio?

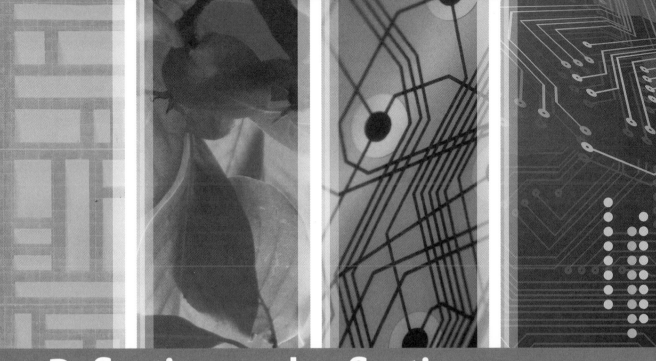

CHAPTER 3

Reflection and reflective practice

Introduction

- You are aware of the requirement to be a reflective practitioner, but how does a portfolio assist in you achieving and demonstrating this?
- What reflective tools might you use to contribute to your portfolio?
- How might you reflect on your overall achievements in order to extend your learning, make a claim of competence, or plan your career?

The purpose of this chapter is to assist readers in understanding and applying reflection techniques in their professional development, learning and portfolio development and use. This will be achieved through a focused overview of the relevant professional literature. As part of this, the meanings and uses of the concept of reflection and the application to the development of portfolios (benefits and tools) for nurses, midwives and other health professionals will be briefly examined. Specific applications to achieving and demonstrating the application and use of reflective skills as a professional achievement will also be included. It is anticipated that this text will assist you in selecting (or possibly

Nursing and Midwifery Portfolios. DOI: 10.1016/B978-0-7295-4078-0.10003-1

developing your own) reflective approaches relevant to the activity you wish to undertake. In order to support you in achieving this, the first section of the text will provide the 'big picture' of the meaning and uses of reflection within professional practice and the relationship between reflection and learning.

Reflection: Meaning and uses within professional practice, learning and portfolios

As Taylor (2006, p. 8) explains, the term reflection within the physical context refers to the 'throwing back from a surface', such as the reflection of heat or sound. When used in the context of human or personal reflection, the term includes not only the re-express — slang for vomiting of thoughts and memories, and hence re-engaging with experiences, but also includes contemplating future actions or change. The complete definition provided by Taylor (2006, p. 8) encapsulates this well when she describes human reflection as: 'throwing back of thoughts and memories, in cognitive acts such as thinking, contemplation, mediation and any other form of attentive consideration, in order to make sense of them, and to make contextually appropriate changes if they are required'.

This definition may be a little confusing initially; however, if we examine its components we can see it is quite useful and achievable. The statement 'throwing back of thoughts and memories' is in effect the process of drawing on past experiences in order to learn from them. Learning from experience, however, is not automatic, nor is it necessarily easy to achieve effectively. You probably have met people whose years of experience do not reflect a high level of personal or extended learning; for example, they may be good at certain tasks but lack the ability to problem solve or understand the perspectives of others. Hence, as Taylor (2006) identifies, reflection requires a level of contemplation or 'cognitive acts' to help broaden and deepen a person's learning. Activities that make us think and reconsider the meaning of events are integral to the reflective process. These can include individual writing activities such as essays and reflective journals, or group interactions such as verbal and written exchanges with a reflective partner or community of practice. Importantly, these are structured in a manner that allows ideas, beliefs and knowledge to be interrogated in order to make sense of a situation and understand it more fully. In doing so we learn to understand both ourselves and the perspectives of others, and to extend our knowledge repertoire through engaging with and applying disciplinary knowledge.

This learning needs to be applied to practice. To do this we need to consider all of the possible solutions and apply the most appropriate one for the specific context. Importantly, reflection on professional practice is not about introspective 'naval gazing'; rather it is about adapting to change and enhancing practice.

This process of drawing on experiences in a deliberate manner in order to enhance our understanding and consider our options for the future has a clear relationship with how we practise in the clinical environment, how we learn in practice, and how we plan and communicate our achievements. Hence the use of the terms 'reflective practice', 'reflective practitioner', 'reflective learning' and 'reflective portfolios' are commonly used in the professional context. Reflective practitioners, for instance, are recognised as individuals who draw on their understanding of how they interact with their environment in order to build upon their knowledge and skills, with the broader objective of enhancing the standard of client care (Jasper 2006). Similarly, the term 'reflective learning' is used to describe the process of drawing on experience to contemplate the meaning, relevance and need for further learning, again with the intent to influence practice standards/ approaches in the future. The analytical aspects of reflection are also necessary when contemplating and framing an argument about competency or other achievements. In order to provide an accurate and substantive argument of achievement, it is necessary to consider or reflect on the evidence of our performance (including omissions in this evidence), contemplate the meaning of the evidence (or lack of it) and frame an argument that communicates and substantiates the conclusions arrived at through the contemplation (André and Heartfield 2007).

As previously indicated, it is the objective of this chapter to support the application of reflection in your professional development, learning and communication of performance outcomes. Portfolios, if used appropriately, are useful tools to assist both in achieving greater levels of reflection and in communicating your achievement of reflective practice and learning. An understanding of the general principles and theoretical assertions that underlie the concepts of reflective practice and reflective learning will assist you in maximising the value of your reflective activities and will be discussed next.

Reflection: Taking a step back, looking at the whole picture, questioning assumptions and considering all options

The various approaches to reflection are based on the premise that we *learn by doing*, and *understanding the impact of our actions* (Dewey, cited in Jasper 2006). Importantly, this learning is not necessarily automatic, as it is a human tendency to want to move quickly to apparently 'easy' single solutions and avoid the hard work of contemplation and questioning. Further, reflective scholars argue that generally our thinking is limited by our unconscious acceptance of cultural 'norms' and values (Dewey, cited in Bulman 2008a). In other words, our view of things is limited by our cultural values and norms and when examining a situation we miss a whole range of possibilities because of this. In short, reflective theory recognises that without supportive scrutiny we do not necessarily understand the impact of what we do, or consider the full range of options we have in changing a situation.

A fundamental aspect of reflective thinking therefore is that we need to find ways of stepping back from situations to examine the full breadth of information, question assumptions and consider the full range of options. On a more personal level, we also need to recognise how our own actions and perceptions may have impacted upon the situation. In addition to needing to acknowledge our contribution to a given situation, reflective writers argue, we also have a responsibility to act on insights we gain through the reflective process, including the need to change our own behaviours (Jasper 2006).

Understanding that the purpose of reflection is to have us consider a situation from a range of perspectives, before jumping ahead to what we think the solution is, is very important in understanding and valuing the reflective process. Consequently, I would very much encourage you to review the following scenario describing a situation when reflective processes are not utilised.

Activity

Reflect upon the following scenario. The questions listed under the headings 'Contemplation stage' and 'Solution stage' have been designed to help you consider the omissions in the reflective process and understand the impact of omissions in the reflective process.

Scenario
Belinda delivers staff development and graduate support programmes at a large metropolitan hospital. At a planning meeting, a nurse manager complains that there is inadequate depth of nursing/midwifery experience to staff the night duty roster. She attributes this to a lack of undergraduate preparation and a failing of the graduate support programme to prepare new graduates for this sort of work early enough. Belinda is given the brief to develop and deliver a staff development session to enable new graduates to work night duty shifts earlier in their employment.

For this exercise we are not disputing the cause attributed to the problems, nor the solution suggested, rather examining the omissions in the reflective process and the impacts this may result in.

Contemplation stage
Do you think that the group gave sufficient attention to contemplating the issues that might have contributed to the lack of staff able to work night duty? Were there other possible causes/issues that needed to be considered before suggesting that new graduates needed to be the solution? *List these here*:

Solution stage

What are the problems in jumping to a single solution in a situation such as this? What other solutions might have been considered? *Detail these here*:

The following are some questions that might otherwise have been asked at the contemplation stage. Compare them with the ones you listed.

· What is the work environment of night duty like? Is it reasonable to expect junior staff to manage in this environment with limited support?
· What sort of skills do staff need to work in this isolated setting?
· How representative is the current staff profile in addressing these needs? Is there some way of providing incentives and support for experienced staff to work night duty?

If these questions were asked then other solutions, such as the following, might have been considered at the solution stage:

· Provide retention incentives for experienced staff to remain on staff.
· Provide incentives for senior staff to work night duty, for instance set rosters and additional holiday relief over school holidays.
· Provide additional supervision support for staff on night duty.

Recall one or more situations you have experienced where limited evidence has been used to justify a supposed solution. How might the outcome have been different if a more reflective approach had been used?

As the above exercise demonstrates, situations where reflective thinking is not used can result in limited and possibly ineffective solutions being proposed. In addition to wasting time and resources, situations such as this can be frustrating to work in and can contribute to an unfulfilling work environment for staff. Many would argue that workplaces that support reflective thinking and analysis are more sustainable due to greater staff satisfaction and productivity (Jasper 2006, Kitchener et al 2006, Taylor 2006, Bulman 2008a).

Summary points

· It is human nature to want to jump to a single solution without considering all the issues and questioning social norms.
· Reflection is a deliberate and structured process of drawing on past events to understand what has happened and question otherwise accepted norms, in order to consider a range of possible actions prior to selecting the most appropriate action for the specific situation.
· Reflection is the basis of reflective practice, reflective learning and career/professional development planning.

What makes a reflective practitioner?

The requirement for reflective practice is well embedded in Australian nursing and midwifery regulation, with references made to reflection or reflective practice in the Competency Standards for Registered Nurses (ANMC 2008a) and Midwives (ANMC 2008b) and in the associated codes of conduct (ANMC 2008c, d). Importantly, reflective practice requires that nurses and midwives are accountable for their current and future actions and therefore need to develop and extend upon their knowledge and skills in response the current and future needs of their clients (Jasper 2006). Further from this, it is this professional accountability that enables nursing and midwifery to be recognised as self-regulated professions, whereby the regulatory authority is drawn from the profession as opposed to a government regulator (Bryant 2005). As the Royal College of Nursing Australia (2006) argues, self-regulation is the aim of any professional group as it enables the profession to set, support and monitor professional standards that address the needs of the public. In order to do this, practitioners first need to be able to account for their own practice and thus develop the necessary skills that will contribute to the continued development of their chosen profession. An important aspect of self-regulation is having practitioners understand their profession and their responsibilities in maintaining and extending professional standards. This starts at the personal level and is the basis of the continuing professional development (CPD) requirement that individual nurses and midwives are accountable for managing their professional development needs (Nursing and Midwifery Board of Australia 2010).

A defining feature of reflective practice is the use of deliberate and considered approaches to examine practice and question routines, with the objective of providing quality services. Individual accountability extends beyond the need to be able to understand and justify current actions, to include responding to change and planning for the future. In order to do this individuals need to reflect upon the current and future healthcare provision and needs of their client group and then have the skills to identify their learning needs, access relevant learning resources and apply the outcomes of learning to practice. There is evidence that the sense of self-determination and professional control associated with reflection supports workplace satisfaction, self-confidence and workplace integrity (Jasper 2006).

In order to respond and improve client care, reflective practitioners need to apply a combination of formal or theoretical knowledge, process skills and personal understandings (Benner et al 2010). Formal knowledge is discipline and specialty-specific knowledge, such as that relating to nursing and midwifery. Discipline-based knowledge is continually developing and expanding through research and professional initiatives such as the development of standards of practice. It is the responsibility of all professionals to keep themselves informed of changes in their disciplinary knowledge through engaging with relevant journals and other recently published works, professional conferences and other professional development activities. As Chapter 4 details, portfolio evidence and arguments need to demonstrate a commitment to contemporary and evidence-based practice in order to be acceptable.

Process skills are necessary in order effectively to access, utilise and evaluate disciplinary knowledge. Process knowledge and skills have been defined as 'knowing how to conduct the various processes that contribute to professional action' (Eraut 2003, p. 107). Clinical reasoning, problem-solving, teamwork, research and communication skills are all forms of process skills (Benner et al 2010). Process skills have commonly been referred to as 'generic skills' because they are a skill set that is shared by all professionals. For instance, the discipline knowledge may differ between nurses, midwives and other health professions; however, skills such as problem-solving, communication and teamwork are a necessary professional skill independent of discipline. The higher education sector is increasingly aware of the need for these skills, and consequently pays considerable attention to the development of what they call 'graduate qualities' or 'graduate attributes' (Barrie & Smith 2009).

In order to practice effectively as professionals, we also need to understand ourselves and how we contribute to or influence outcomes and situations (Norman 2008). For instance, professionals have a responsibility to understand and manage how they best learn, what motivates them to perform well and how they react in given situations. As various professional codes of conduct and ethics illustrate, there is a professional requirement for nurses and midwives to understand themselves and to manage their professional situations such that they provide high levels of care and do not negatively impact upon the rights and care of individuals (ANMC 2008c, d, e). For instance, a nurse or midwife has the right not to participate in an activity on religious or moral grounds, but also has a responsibility to do so in a manner that does not impact on the rights of others (ANMC 2008e). In order to do this it is therefore necessary for individuals to prepare themselves by reflecting on their personal beliefs, and consider how best to manage professional situations that might cause them conflict. This conflict need not be the 'big ticket' ethical items such as termination of pregnancy procedure; it also includes 'everyday ethics' such as managing and reporting situations of concern (Benner et al 2010). For instance, a person may know how to manage conflict or understand the need to report suspected child abuse, but this does not necessarily mean that they will act on this knowledge when the need arises. Importantly, professionals need to have considered their ethical values, motivations and other forms of self-understanding in order to ensure that they are in the best situation to provide quality care, in both the short and long term.

As has been explained above, reflective and accountable practice is the essence of professionalism and supports the underpinnings of professional self-regulation. Reflective practitioners use deliberate and considered approaches to examine their practice and question otherwise taken-for-granted routines and practices in order to enact effective change, both in the short and long term. It is through individuals reflecting on, and using, their formal knowledge, process skills and self-understanding that they actively develop and expand on their knowledge and skills to support improvements in client care. While this may sound like an obvious process, the achievement and application of reflective professionalism is quite complex. Learning activities such as student portfolios, reflective journals and self-assessment exercises are used as part of undergraduate education programmes to assist students progressively to acquire, apply and understand the necessary skills to become a reflective practitioner.

How does this relate to reflective learning?

There are a range of ways in which learning can be explained and supported. Reflection and 'reflective learning theory' is a particularly useful approach for clinical practice as it recognises that people make sense of their learning through application and considering the impact of their actions. This section of the chapter will provide an overview of reflective learning theory and how this might be used in professional practice using the experiential learning approach developed by David Kolb (1984) and others.

It is through practice-based experience, and associated reflections that people make sense of how meaningful some learning is, based on how useful it is to them in practice (Taylor 2006). For instance, in undergraduate education it is common to study conflict resolution techniques and use role-play to practise these in the classroom. However, it is not until a range of conflict situations are experienced that the value of this learning is often understood.

It is the need to act in new or difficult situations that can motivate careful examination of potential conflict and bring to light some of the things that inform the choice of resolution approaches. Like most learning, insights about behaviour and options occur over time and with the support and critique of colleagues, mentors and friends.

It is important to reiterate that reflection within the professional context is not limited to introspective reflections about our actions, rather it is an important tool/stimulus for changing behaviours (Taylor 2006). As Bulman (2008a, p. 2) also reminds us, an important part of reflection is opening up our practice for others to examine, and 'consequently requires courage and

open-mindedness as well as willingness to take on board and act on criti-
cism'. Hence, activities such as performance reviews or peer assessment
processes should be enacted as potentially important learning opportunities.
It is tempting to be discouraged or avoid situations that threaten us;
however, considerable professional growth is achieved by engaging with,
and reflecting on, these challenges.

As many of the reflective learning scholars affirm, experience informs
learning. As Donald Schön (1983), for example, explains, it is a process of
reflection both during and after experiences that enables practitioners to
extend from single focus rule driven behaviours to understanding the
context or 'big picture' of a situation, and its associated causes and conse-
quences. Schön explains that this ability to manage and understand
complexity and uncertainty does not happen because of a single event.
Rather, the skills of reflection need to start initially as a conscious and
deliberate activity, but with practice within the applied work environment,
become an unconscious automatic process (Schön 1987). As mentioned
earlier, this learning occurs over time, with repeated exposures and
continued effort.

As both Schön (1983, 1987) and Patricia Benner (Benner 1984, Benner et al
2010) explain, with repeated and frequent use reflective thinking can
become an automatic process that occurs without conscious effort. For this
reason, some expert practitioners find it difficult to explain how they arrived
at a decision, as they are not necessarily aware of the intuitive reflective
processes that inform their actions. This is not to say that they do not use
reflective thinking, rather reflection becomes so much part of their everyday
practice that it is unremarkable and an unconscious act unless there is cause
to stop and reconstruct the thinking that informed their actions. Consequently, it is often difficult for students and other less experienced staff to
observe how experts use reflective thinking, particularly in situations that
require quick action. Hence, the use of deliberate learning activities, such as
critical incident analysis, are important in understanding and learning from
experts (Taylor 2006).

Learning from experience and developing reflective skills in practice is an
important requirement in becoming an expert practitioner (Benner 1984).
A useful learning theory to support learning within and from experience has
been developed by David Kolb, in what is referred to as 'experiential learning'
(Kolb 1984). Experiential learning is an approach that enables individuals and
others to recognise formal and non-formal learning within a practice context.
As Pearce (2003) identifies, the values of Kolb's model of experiential
learning, whereby links are made between formal learning, workplace
learning and personal development, reflect the important principles that
portfolios represent. It is therefore useful to understand the principles and
practices of experiential learning, in order to best utilise your portfolio. For
this reason, this approach will be elaborated upon more fully here.

Experiential learning examined

The premise of experiential learning is that quality learning is achieved via using experience as a basis of reflection and application. As in the much quoted words of the Chinese philosopher Confucius (551–479 BC), 'tell me and I will forget, show me and I may remember, involve me and I will understand' (Wang 2004, p. 64). The need to be involved in order to understand, and the importance of this to deep and applied learning, has clearly been well understood for some time. It is through this deep and applied learning that students and practitioners understand the consequence and rationales of their actions. A useful indicator that quality learning has occurred is being able demonstrate skills in a practice environment and explain:

· the reasons for the actions undertaken
· the intended outcomes of the action
· the alternatives considered when deciding on the best way to proceed
· the potential repercussions that would be monitored for.

The above explanations are probably familiar to most of us as these are common questions that supervising staff are likely to ask students or novices in the clinical environment. Assessing for applied understanding is important both to stimulate this deeper learning and to ensure the provision of safe and professional practice in changing circumstances. As a consequence, experiential learning, and hence these sorts of questions, are commonly used in clinical learning environments.

Experiential learning is based on the following principles:

· For learning to be meaningful it must result in changes to practice and behaviours.
· By seeing the value and impact of our learning we are motivated to learn further.
· Quality learning can be achieved equally in formal and informal learning environments once an individual has developed effective learning skills.
· Individuals need to be open and ready to learn, this requires us to be able to engage in self-critique, feedback and be prepared to change our behaviours.
· Learning is enhanced in supportive environments that encourage honesty, respect and value innovation and change (Jasper 2006).

There are several depictions of the experiential learning model, each explaining a cycle of events that includes some form of experience, reflection and application to practice. The one shown in Figure 3.1 is commonly associated with Kolb, but he himself gives credit to Kurt Lewin for the basic design (Kolb 1984, p. 21).

As Kolb identifies, reflection is an effective approach for recognising and integrating formal learning with informal learning though practice. In order to achieve this, the learner needs to reflect on their practice/experience in

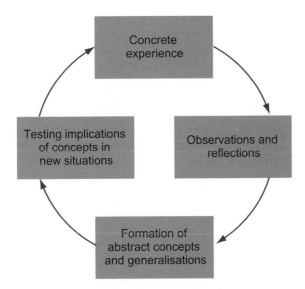

FIGURE 3.1 The Lewinian experiential learning model (Kolb 1984, p. 21)

a considered manner in order to support the formation of a conceptual understanding that can be generalised beyond the specific experience. This concept then needs to be tested/attempted in practice, and this application of theory to practice then provides a further concrete experience to reflect upon (Kolb 1984). The relationship between practice application and theoretical concepts is an important one for professional learning, as conceptual frameworks enable the generalisation of knowledge beyond single specific incidences. While it may be appropriate to train semi-skilled workers to follow task lists, the very nature of a professional role requires a level of understanding to support the ability to predict and respond to change.

The following activity has been designed to help you understand how the experiential learning model might be used in practice.

Activity

Reflect on the following scenario and identify the four components in the model, namely

1. concrete experience
2. observation and reflection
3. abstract concept and generalisation
4. testing implications of concepts in new situations.

Scenario

Deborah is a 24-year-old woman who has recently had her first baby. Belinda, the midwife caring for her, notices that Deborah is very agitated when dealing with her baby. In one instance, Belinda was called away while Deborah was bathing her baby. When Belinda returned she found the baby naked in its cot and Deborah in her bed saying she had become panicky, dizzy and unable to breathe. Later when she had recovered, Deborah explained that she had felt like this before when presented with stressful situations. She explained that she had previously managed her anxiety by removing herself from the situation for a few minutes, and that she was usually able to 'gather herself together' and deal with the situation. Deborah explained that she could manage most emergency situations and that her behaviour was 'no big deal'. She specifically asked Belinda not mention it to anyone as she said she was able to manage.

That evening Belinda reviewed the literature about anxiety disorders and panic attacks and noted that Deborah was showing many of the clinical features. As part of this reading, Belinda also noted that there is a co-morbid relationship between anxiety disorders and depression, with a considerable overlap in the clinical features. When considering a course of action, Belinda reflected on her limited role and experience in diagnosing and treating psychological disorders, but also understood that if Deborah did suffer from a form of anxiety or depression and if left untreated, her condition could worsen, with potentially serious implications.

Within her reading, Belinda also noted that those with anxiety disorders often felt they were being scrutinised and judged by others, and that an important part of the treatment was to enable individuals to overcome their fears in a supportive and non-judgemental environment. Therefore she decided to proceed carefully, trying to involve Deborah in the decision-making process, thus maintaining her trust and setting the scene for a therapeutic relationship with her in the future. The next day Belinda spent time with Deborah gently explaining the benefits of early assessment and intervention in situations such as hers. Deborah agreed to see a clinical psychologist and they were able to make an appointment for the following day.

Reflections

Concrete experience
Observation and reflection
Abstract concept and generalisation
Testing implications of concepts in new situations

While there is no absolute correct answer as to the components of the experiential learning model within the above scenario, the following are my reflections on this scenario:

There is some overlap between the *concrete experience* of this scenario (Belinda observing Deborah's behaviours) and the *observation and reflection* (talking to Deborah after the bathing event and reflecting on this and information from the literature). Belinda's review of the literature that evening allowed her to engage in further reflection in order to move into the *formation of abstract concepts and generalisations*, namely conceptualising:

· the need to act due to the potential seriousness of the situation
· the need to act in a manner that would enhance self-determination and trust and thus support future therapy.

Speaking to Deborah the following day was a form of *testing the implications of these concepts in new situations*; in particular, Belinda enacted a trusting and supportive relationship with her client in order to further her care. This then forms the next *concrete experience* and commences the cycle again.

As has been discussed in this section, reflective learning is an important part of professional learning and development as the focus is on changing and enhancing practice. The experiential learning model is a useful reflective framework to guide professional learning, as a central tenet is the integration of formal learning and application to practice. Importantly, by using practice to understand what we need to learn, and to understand the relevance of our learning, we are able to direct and justify our professional development needs, and hence act in a self-determining and professionally extending manner.

Summary Points

· Reflective practitioners are accountable for the current and future care they provide, and therefore need to examine their practice and question routines, with the objective of providing quality services.
· Clinical knowledge is a combination of theoretical knowledge, process skills and personal understandings.
· It is through practice-based experience, and associated reflections, that people make sense of how meaningful some learning is, based on how useful it is to them in practice.
· Reflection is initially a conscious and deliberate activity, but with practice becomes an unconscious, automatic process embedded in expert practice.
· The experiential learning model is an approach used by novice clinicians to develop reflective skills through applying a structured framework of drawing on concrete experiences to observe and reflect, formulate abstract concepts and then test the implications of these concepts in new situations.

Tools for reflection

The requirement for nurses, midwives and other professions to be self-directed and accountable for their professional development is integral to regulatory requirements both in Australia (Nursing and Midwifery Board of Australia 2010) and internationally. Employers are responsible for providing opportunities for their staff to undertake their continued professional development; however, a responsibility of each professional to identify and prioritise their learning needs, develop their own learning plan and reflect on the value of the activities undertaken (Nursing and Midwifery Board of Australia 2010).

As has been discussed in Chapter 1, portfolios provide a useful educational tool to document and develop professional development processes, as well as other reflective learning and application processes. As a reminder, a quality portfolio is all of the following:

· a storage space(collection of artefacts)
· a workspace (collection plus reflection)
· a showcase (selection, summative reflection and presentation) (Barrett 2007).

Importantly, reflection is what 'makes' a portfolio. Without the reflective component, a portfolio is merely a 'work log' or basic curriculum vitae (Jasper 2006). The reflective aspect allows you to create a whole story about your achievements, drawing on work-related issues through journals, demonstrating the application of discipline knowledge and process skills though care plans, and demonstrating insight and self-understanding through action plans, etc. (Pearce 2003). Importantly portfolio activities and showcasing enable you to generalise from specific experiences to claim competence for both past and future professional activities. The real value of a portfolio lies in the reflection and learning that are generated from the activities, including the meta-cognitive act of framing an argument of achievement that draws on the various recorded activities (Barrett 2009). It is through this reflection and integration of formal and informal learning that portfolios enhance links between education, work and personal development and make processes associated with accountability and responsibility of care more apparent and meaningful.

Reflective tools, either within the portfolio framework or independently accessed, are particularly important in introducing and structuring reflection for both novice practitioners and experienced staff. As previously indicated, it is human nature to want to skip the assessment and contemplation stages of reflection and grab at a single but appealing answer. It is therefore important that all professionals consider using reflective tools to structure the process and challenge habitual thinking (Jasper 2006).

All reflective activities/tools have some or all of the following components:

· draw on some form of experience; this can be formal learning, workplace experience or similar
· use a framework to support you in describing the experience from various perspectives, critically analysing it to question your assumptions and 'challenge habitual thinking'
· conceptualise/map ideas and develop a systematic plan of how and what is to be implemented
· implement the plan, apply ideas to practice and evaluate the impact (Taylor 2006).

So what is the best tool/approach to use? There is an array of reflective tools used in education and practice, each with differing qualities and contexts of use. Broad approaches, such as the experiential learning model explained earlier, are particularly useful in structuring and reflecting learning activities. Other more focused approaches support more specific outcomes, such as structured personal reflections, critical incident analysis or the development of a learning plan. It is important to understand the basic intent of various approaches and select or develop an appropriate tool for your specific task.

As you develop your reflection skills, you will need to draw on a range of tools and approaches in order to demonstrate a breadth of skills and achievements. To select the most appropriate approach for an activity, you might like to consider the following:

· What is the purpose of this reflective activity in this specific situation?
· What resources do I have to achieve the purpose?
· How will I know if I have a quality product at the end?

There are many reasons for reflection; however, for the most part the purpose of a reflective activity will include some or all of the following:

· support effective learning that incorporates questioning practices, considering a range of options and implementing a possible solution
· learn from clinical situations
· consider how best to apply formal learning outcomes to practice
· plan your learning needs, performance review or career plan
· engage others in evaluating or developing your practice.

A range of tools according to each of these categories has been included later in this chapter. For the time being, however, it is important to consider the conditions necessary to assist you to learn through reflection. These include:

· Preparation — be prepared to engage in opportunities for reflection. Initially this might feel contrived and awkward; however, with practice you will come to see the benefits and the process becomes easier.
· Understanding — you need to understand the goals and expectations of reflection, namely to contemplate given situations in order to 1) better

understand the situation and taken for granted assumptions, 2) consider all options and 3) act upon the outcomes.

· Time — give yourself time to stop, think and reflect on situations.
· Objectivity and honesty — you need to develop an objective stance where you step back from your interpretations of situations and be honest about your influence and the impact of your actions. It is important to have an open, non-defensive attitude to the experience.
· Deeper levels of meaning — be prepared to consider the deeper meaning of moral, ethical, social and/or professional issues (Branch & Paranjape 2002) in addition to your emotional response (Monash University 2010).

Learning from a clinical/practice situation

It is important to select specific aspects of your practice to reflect upon. In particular, identify situations that are unusual or significant in some way that provide you with a learning opportunity. The significance of a situation might be that it occurs often and needs improvement (frequent and low impact), or that it is an unusual event with major ramifications (infrequent with high impact). Both positive and negative events can provide useful learning situations. Importantly, select a situation that is relevant to your learning. For instance, if you are inexperienced in managing aggressive clients in the workplace, you might choose to focus on an incident which was managed well by a more experienced staff member.

Having selected the situation, you need to select a tool or activity to help with your reflection process. It is important that this is an active process, that provides a record of your reflections. While we may feel comforted that our thoughts and daydreams are well-structured and deeply contemplative, in reality when you try to recall these thoughts you may well find that this has not been the case. The process of writing is a useful way to structure and justify our thinking (Taylor 2006). Writing is a purposeful activity that requires us to focus our attention, order our thoughts and make causal and explanatory connections, thus generating further ideas (Jasper 2006). The permanent record of the written word also assists us to return to these thoughts for the purposes of further extension, or importantly, when constructing a portfolio to be submitted for some form of assessment, to use as evidence of an achievement.

Reflective writing

The following is a basic introduction to reflective writing approaches. There are many high quality texts dedicated to the development of reflective writing skills that extend well beyond the information that appears here (see, for example, Jasper 2006, Taylor 2006, Bulman & Schutz 2008). Most university programmes also include support in how to develop and structure your writing, which may be useful if you require further assistance.

Writing is an interesting process as it focuses and centres our attention and thoughts. For many people, it takes time to appreciate the process of writing, as we can feel threatened by setting down our ideas and work for others to read. However, as professionals, it is important that we engage with the exercise of writing, for it is a very useful tool to help us make contact with our unexamined thoughts and create connections with new information (Jasper 2006). The tangible nature of the written word is part of the benefit of writing reflectively. This allows us to revisit our written work, discuss it with others or use it as evidence in our portfolios.

As Jasper (2006, p. 83) describes, reflective writing is a particular form of writing 'that is done for the purposes of learning' by exploring a subject in depth. While reflective journals are commonly associated with reflective writing, any number of approaches meet this criteria, including formal essays, blog entries or a summary written as part of your clinical performance self-assessment. The various strategies for reflective writing have been described as being on a continuum from highly analytical, such as a critical incident analysis, through to highly creative acts, such as writing poetry (Jasper 2006). It is important that you choose the appropriate approach, one which enables you to achieve the outcome you intend. For instance, a reflective journal is a useful way to understand yourself and how you interact with your professional environment, whereas a 'strengths, weaknesses, opportunities and treats (SWOT)' analysis is more focused towards developing and insti-gating an action plan. The following are a few focused strategies that may assist you in understanding and selecting a reflective writing approach that best suits your task.

Reflective journal or blog entry

As previously mentioned, using a reflective journal can be a useful approach to structure our thoughts about an event or a series of events. Increasingly individuals are using blogs for this purpose, either choosing to keep their online blog entries private, or seeking feedback with a limited or extended audience of blog users. Whether using pen and paper or computer tech-nologies, it is important to consider how to structure your entries to support the reflective process.

There are many ways to construct your reflective journal or online blog entries. The Gibbs reflective cycle has been selected here as it has the benefit of dealing with both events and the feelings that the experience generated (Bulman 2008, Ch. 9). By understanding the feelings we associate with certain situations we are better able to understand how our perceptions are influ-enced by our emotions, and through this understanding we are more likely to be perceptive to the experiences of others. For instance, by understanding how angry we were in a particular situation we are more likely to be able to stop and reflect on the intent of others, and consider that their intent may not have been malicious. Understanding our emotions is, however, not the only focus. The complete Gibbs's reflective cycle is illustrated in Figure 3.2:

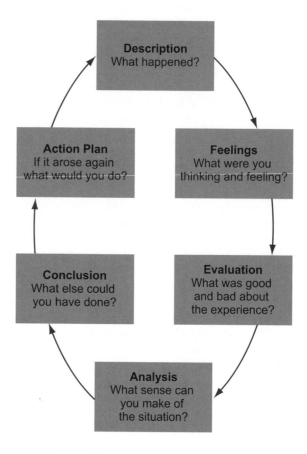

FIGURE 3.2 Gibbs's reflective cycle (Gibbs et al 1988)

When using any reflective approach, it is important to be aware that there are levels of reflection, and deeper levels of reflection will assist us to achieve a more resilient outcome. For instance, when using the above reflective cycle, it is important to consider the following:

·   When recording your *description* of the event, refrain from making judgements or reaching conclusions; rather describe the events as objectively as you can.
·   Similarly, in the *feelings* component, force yourself to describe how you felt and focus on this before moving to the evaluation and analysis component. Also include in here how others might have felt.
·   In the *evaluation* section, list all the positive and negative aspects of the experience. This is important to put the event into perspective and assists those who are at risk of over- or under-reacting to a situation.

- The *analysis* section is where you start to make sense of the situation. Contemplate all the possible causes or impacting variables that may have contributed to the situation. Do not limit yourself to the one you think is most likely, but consider all the alternatives. Past experiences, literature or other external sources may be of use here.
- As part of the *conclusion*, consider the likely issues that contributed to the situation and range of actions you or others might have done that would have changed the situation.
- From this, you can develop your *action plan*. What would you do differently if this situation were to happen again? And, how might you prepare yourself for this? Again, do not limit your options until you have considered all possibilities and selected the most achievable and effective plan (Bulman 2008, Ch. 9).

Activity

Select a recent significant experience and use Gibbs reflective cycle to record and reflect upon the incident. It is recommended that you choose an experience that was very emotionally charged and significant to you. Take your time to work through the following reflective process, ensuring that you record as many details as possible. A series of questions have been included to act as prompts to help you.

Description

> What did I do?
> What did others do?
> What happened next?

Feelings

> How did I feel?
> How might others have felt?

Evaluation

> What was I trying to achieve?
> What was good about this experience?
> What was bad about this experience/event?

Analysis

> What are the various explanations for what happened here?
> How might the events have appeared from others' perspective?
> Having read the literature about this topic, what other explanations are there for what happened here?

Conclusions

> Having reviewed all the possibilities, what are the likely issues that contributed to this situation?

What range of actions might you or others have done that would have changed the situation?

Action plan

What would I do differently if this situation were to happen again? How might I prepare myself for this?

What outcomes will I demonstrate that indicate that I have achieved this action plan?

Having completed the above reflection, provide a brief summary of your use of the Gibbs reflective cycle.

Did you find that the structured approach helped to draw out information that you might not have considered?

What were the limitations of this process for you?

How useful was this exercise in having you distance yourself from the situation and understand the perspective of others?

Are some of the components of your action plan an extension of what you would ordinarily have learnt for this situation without the use of a reflective cycle?

Critical incident analysis

A critical incident analysis is a focused reflective activity about an incident that had meaning and learning potential. While it is common to focus on negative incidents, this need not necessarily be the case, as much can also be learnt from 'getting something right'. The analysis activity can be undertaken as a group activity, a written paper or a blog/journal entry. There are various formats or frameworks used to deconstruct and analyse an incident, including Gibbs reflective cycle (Gibbs et al 1988), mentioned earlier. Whatever approach used, it is important to ask yourself questions such as:

· How might others have perceived this situation?
· Why did I interpret the situation as I did?
· Have I considered all the possible reasons for this situation having occurred as it did?
· What are all of the possible actions that could have helped in this situation?
· What would I do in a similar situation in the future and how might I prepare myself?

The following is the approach of recording a critical incident analysis used at Monash University (2010). It includes useful information about the language that should be used in order to draw on the necessary information.

Scenario — Example critical incident analysis

Context of the Incident

This report will outline a critical incident which occurred in Week 9, Semester 2 in my clinical tutorial. The incident was initiated by my tutor, who announced that she would provide individual feedback to students on their performance in clinical tutorial discussions. She also stated that she would be producing written comments on each student's behaviour, attitude and contribution in tutorials to be incorporated into student portfolios for Semester 2.

Details of the Incident

At the end of my clinical tutorial my tutor arranged for us to meet briefly in order for her to discuss her feedback with me. She stated that over the semester she had noticed that I very rarely spoke in the tutorials and did not appear to engage with the other students. She was concerned that I appeared to lack confidence, and explained that being able to express opinions clearly and confidently was essential in my future career as a doctor. In her view the only way to develop confidence was to partic-ipate regularly. She asked me how I felt about this, and if there was a reason why I almost never spoke in class. I explained that in my culture students were not always encouraged to speak, and for that reason I did not find it easy. I also mentioned that I sometimes feel shy.

Note the use of first person to describe the writer's reactions and feelings:

> I explained …
> I mentioned …
> I felt embarrassed …
> I was worried that …
> I realised that …

Note the use of reported speech to describe the conversations between those involved in the incident.

> She stated that …
> She was concerned that …
> In her view …

Thoughts, Feelings and Concerns

At the time of this incident, many emotions were running through me. I felt embarrassed that my lack of confidence was so obvious to her, and also concerned about what impact it might have on my results. I was worried that she would write negative comments about my behaviour and atti-tude, and that these comments would be available for other lecturers to read. At the same time, I realised that her concerns were justified — I had been aware of my lack of contribution throughout the semester, and had even avoided going to some tutorials because of those feelings. This was also an unfamiliar situation for me, as I had always done very well at school and achieved good marks, so I had never had to talk with a teacher in this way before. Although I understood that her intention was to help me to do better, I felt very uncomfortable and even ashamed to have to acknowledge my poor performance in this area. I felt guilty when I realised that in her opinion I had contributed so little to the class.

Demands

This incident was very demanding because it forced me to acknowledge an area where I have always lacked confidence. Even though I preferred to focus on other areas, I knew that my tutor would be noticing my behaviour in tutorials over the rest of the semester, and that her written comments would depend on my performance, so as a consequence I felt under pressure. I also felt anxious about confronting this issue and trying to develop the confidence I needed.

Impact on Studies

Although this incident caused me discomfort and added pressure in the short term, I realise that it was a very significant event in my studies. As a result of the conversation with my tutor I was forced to reconsider my behaviour in tutorials and became more aware of how others viewed me. I had been used to think that I was 'invisible' in tutorials, but now I realised that not talking actually made me stand out more. Fortunately, the tutor gave me advice on how gradually to develop the confidence I needed, and I also sought help from some of my friends. I even organised to have some informal tutorials with friends to give me a chance to practise. Over the final weeks of the semester I managed to talk at least once in every clinical tutorial, either asking a question or making a comment. I have started trying to talk in other tutorials also, in other subjects. I have set myself the goal of talking at least once every tutorial.

This incident was therefore very important, because without it I would still be remaining silent in my tutorials, and would have received negative written comments from my clinical tutor in my portfolio. More importantly, it has helped me to acknowledge and work on an area for improvement which will be beneficial in all aspects of the course. Developing greater confidence at speaking in tutorials may lead to my being more confident in performing clinical examinations on patients. It may also lead to me feeling more in control and experiencing less nerves during my Objective Structured Clinical Examination (OSCE) assessments.

Impact on Career

My tutor was right in stating that a doctor must be able to express opinions clearly and confidently. Good communication skills are essential for doctors, and are important in nearly all aspects of medicine. I feel that I will be more confident in dealing with patients and more effective in taking a patient history, for example. Developing greater confidence in how I communicate can lead to patients having greater trust in me as their doctor. Improving my skills in this area will also make me more effective in discussing cases with colleagues, and in participating in teams when necessary.

This incident made me realise that I can talk confidently once I overcome my initial fears. It demonstrated to me that in order to make progress or create positive change you must first acknowledge that a problem exists. This is a lesson which may be useful in better understanding patient behaviour and attitudes. Often the first step to improving a situation, or dealing with a problem, is accepting that some change is necessary; and I may be more able to impart this information to patients having experienced this incident. Overall, this incident has had a positive impact on both my studies and on the development of skills needed in my future career.

(Monash University 2010).

Source: http://www.monash.edu.au/lls/llonline/writing/medicine/reflective/5.xml, accessed 2010. Reproduced with permission from Monash University Library.

Concept maps

An important aspect of reflection is the ability to conceptualise or map ideas. A concept map is a diagrammatic representation of the relationships between information and is used to structure and communicate the assimilation of clusters of information within a 'big picture' image. The basic premise of concept maps is that understanding is enhanced by relating information in a meaningful way (Schuster 2008). When developing a concept map, information is clustered into like groups and then presented pictorially to illustrate how these component groupings relate to the whole. You might be familiar with concept maps that appear as illustrations or figures within textbooks or as a slide within lectures. These maps are a useful way to illustrate the various components of a pathophysiological or other process. In most instances, concept maps are accompanied by a written or verbal explanation detailing the meaning of the illustration. The concept map provides a useful visual summary, making it a useful teaching tool. Figure 3.3 illustrates the nursing process and is an example of a simple concept map. As those of you who are familiar with the nursing process will be aware, it gives a deceptively simplified version of what is quite a technically difficult process in practice. The simplification and pictorial depiction of the process, however, provides us with a useful learning framework to structure and inform the practice application.

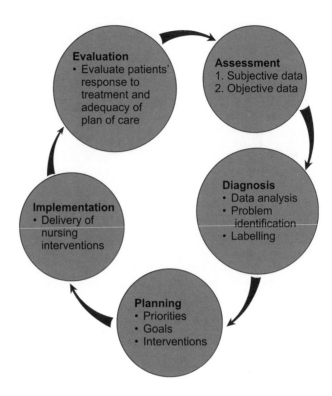

FIGURE 3.3 The nursing process

In addition to providing a useful 'end' picture, the process of developing a concept map is a useful method of helping us to link new and existing information (Gaberson & Oermann 2007). Concept maps have been used to prepare care plans, for example, to conceptualise the links between the pathophysiology of a condition and the rationales of care, or to structure idea generation exercises such as 'brainstorming' activities (Schuster 2008). Using concept maps as a method of reviewing and summarising your learning is a useful technique to prepare for exams as if used well the process requires the student to engage with the content, and the map itself is a useful summary and revision tool.

The process of using a concept map to structure ideas and thinking includes the following stages:

· purpose identification and clarification
· idea/information generation
· idea/information clustering
· structuring a hierarchy of clusters.

The following demonstrates the use of concept maps to design and write complex articles, such as this chapter, to elaborate on the four stages listed

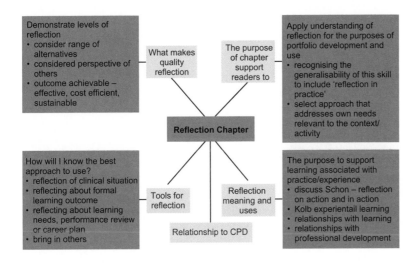

Demonstrate levels of
reflection
• consider range of
  alternatives
• considered perspective of
  others
• outcome achievable –
  effective, cost efficient,
  sustainable

What makes
quality
reflection

The purpose
of chapter
support
readers to

Apply understanding of
reflection for the purposes of
portfolio development and
use
• recognising the
  generalisability of this skill
  to include 'reflection in
  practice'
• select approach that
  addresses own needs
  relevant to the context/
  activity

Reflection Chapter

How will I know the best
approach to use?
• reflection of clinical situation
• reflecting about formal
  learning outcome
• reflecting about learning
  needs, performance review
  or career plan
• bring in others

Tools for
reflection

Reflection
meaning and
uses

The purpose to support
learning associated with
practice/experience
• discuss Schon – reflection
  on action and in action
• Kolb experientail learning
• relationships with learning
• relationships with
  professional development

Relationship to CPD

FIGURE 3.4 A concept map for the development of this chapter

above. *Clarifying the purpose* of a concept mapping exercise prior to
commencing is important in order to maintain the focus of the exercise. If
a mapping exercise does not work, it is usually because the purpose of the
exercise is confused or unclear. As a consequence a purpose statement is
included within the map as this helped clarify thinking and justify the
inclusion and structuring of materials. As you will note in the concept map in
Figure 3.4, the purpose statement is written as a performance outcome or
objective that explains 'what is hoped to achieve within this article'. Having
settled on a purpose statement, the salient points are recorded. During
this idea generation stage, all manner of ideas and sources, including
reviewing the literature, are considered including colleagues' opinions and
'brainstorming' outcomes. It is important to note that this stage can be quite
lengthy as it is important to consider a range of approaches and ideas prior to
setting out a plan. Bring together new ideas from readings and record these
on a concept map with a code that records where the idea came from. Over
time, numerous isolated items of information are collected. As links start to
emerge, arrows can be drawn between items, but avoid clustering information until as many new ideas as possible are recorded. When no new ideas
come to light it is time to develop the plan. At this stage examine the relevance of various items and cluster them into groups. These clusters are groups
of information about the same topic. By progressively moving between the
purpose statement and the information clusters, the overall plan or map is
formulated. This is the point at which to develop a hierarchical structure that
explains how each of the clusters relates to each other with the overall intent
of addressing the purpose statement. The diagram in Figure 3.4 with
major headings and subheadings is in effect the plan used to write this
chapter.

The figure is a simplified version of the final map that illustrates the original hierarchical structuring for this chapter. Note the final chapter varies from this; however, the map provided an important beginning structure and allowed more detailed writing.

While the task of writing a full book chapter is particularly complex, and so a specialised software program is very useful, it is possible to use a similar process for smaller activities with a whiteboard or A3 paper.

The following activity draws on a concept map activity recently used as a staff development exercise in applying the NMBA Nursing and Midwifery Continuing Professional Development Registration Standard (Nursing and Midwifery Board of Australia 2010). The purpose of this mapping exercise was to have the participants use the AMNC competency statements to consider the full range of possible staff learning needs within the context of their organisation. Participants were provided with the concept map structure, and asked to 'brainstorm' according to each of the various categories. The reflective nature of this exercise was important in having the participants think of a range of ideas before focusing on priorities or being limited by pragmatics of what staff development opportunities already existed.

Activity

The purpose of the following exercise is for you to develop a list of possible learning needs for someone working as a registered nurse or registered midwife in your workplace (or most recent clinical placement environment if you are a student). While not part of this activity, the intention of this exercise is that this list would assist you in formulating your learning priorities and thus contribute to your annual CPD learning plan.

To complete this specific activity, for three of the competency headings, list as many relevant learning issues that relate to:

· your current position description (if you are planning to apply for a promotion or position change in the near future, you might also want to include those relevant to this)
· the specific clinical environment
· changing client demographic and disease/health profiles (e.g. changes in socio-cultural or illness profile of those attending this healthcare facility)
· healthcare priorities for your institution.

For instance, under the heading of 'Practices in accordance with legislation' list the legislation relevant to your RN/RM position description/role that are significant to this clinical environment. For example, a nurse manager may include aspects of industrial legislation that has less relevance to a staff member working as a level 1 RN/RM. The clinical context will also influence the relevance of some legislation, for instance a more detailed understanding of legislation about elder abuse or food safety will be relevant to the aged care sector. Completing all ten competency items will obviously be time consuming, so for the time being you might want to choose three. If you find this exercise useful, you might want to have your colleagues help you to complete the full concept map (Figure 3.5). This list would also be relevant to any of them.

Having listed all the possible areas for at least three competency headings, mark an asterisk next to each item on the basis of each of the following:

· recent changes in this area (new policies, legislation or equipment)
· an area of personal weakness
· an area of increasing clinical significance (e.g. changes to your client population demographics or disease profiles)
· a deficit in this area has resulted in a significant clinical incident in the recent past
· a significant milestone necessary for your promotion
· a set of skills needed for emergencies
· other relevant priorities.

Review those items marked with asterisks and list at least three learning priorities for the forthcoming year.

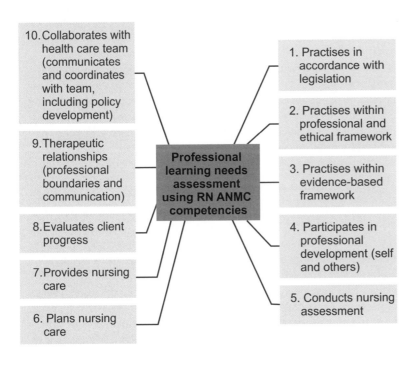

FIGURE 3.5 Beginning concept map for assessing learning needs against ANMC competencies

How useful was this exercise in generating a broader range of ideas that you might not have otherwise considered?

Engaging others

Engaging others in our reflections is an important strategy in broadening our perspective and gauging our own performance as compared with our peer group. Having said this, not everyone is ready to receive critique, nor will all our colleagues give the level and quality of critique necessary to assist us. There are times when we have some level of choice in whom we can call upon to help us with our reflection, for instance if setting up a mentoring programme, developing an online community of practice or structuring a professional reflection group. There are, however, times when our choice of those we are able to include as part of our reflective activity is limited; for instance, generally we have little say in the appointment of our clinical supervisor or who will manage our performance appraisal process. Whatever the situation, the skills of giving and receiving feedback are very significant in making the most of these opportunities.

Why engage with others?

Having others critique and contribute to our work has the potential to expand and advance the outcome significantly. A well structured group/relationship can assist in motivation, efficiency and the overall quality of the product of the group endeavour. Groups working together have been shown to produce more significant outcomes than if the same activity were undertaken by individuals. In other words, there are significant potential benefits in sharing your reflections and working with others to assist in your development. Groups can, however, also be ineffective, or worse, destructive to individuals. Hence it is important to instigate strategies to support the development of positive group dynamics when setting up your peer appraisal activity, online blog or mentoring programme.

How to engage others

It is important when setting up a peer support or appraisal process that the right individuals are involved and that the 'rules of engagement' are clear and well understood. The 'right individuals' are those able and willing to critique your work and help you to develop strategies to develop professionally. You will need to make your own judgement about individuals who best meet these criteria. In some instances, your line manager or peers may have these requisite skills while in other situations you might be better off having someone from outside your institution provide a 'fresh perspective' to your reflections. Whatever the situation it is important to choose carefully and be clear about what you hope to achieve from the relationship.

As previously mentioned, setting the 'rules of engagement' early is also important. The following points are the sorts of details that should be discussed with your mentor at your first meeting:

· purpose and duration of the arrangement, including time commitments required
· sorts of activities to be undertaken, e.g. case study reviews, debriefing exercises, etc.
· preparation commitments for each meeting, e.g. will you be setting an agenda, providing a written reflection to discuss, etc.
· confidentiality of information exchanged
· commitment to honest and productive processes, including being open to change
· a clarification of boundaries, for instance mentoring roles should not interfere with other professional relationships.

It is important to discuss the specifics of each of these to support a shared understanding of what these mean in practice.

An important part of engaging with others in a professional and effective manner is our commitment to providing and receiving quality feedback. Quality feedback is appropriately timed, descriptive and specific, constructive and tailored to the individual. 'Appropriately timed' can, of course, mean different things to different people; however, for the most part it means as soon as practical following the incident or episode, while taking into account the need for discretion. Descriptive, specific and constructive feedback provides the individual with a balance of sufficient details to make a more general point, while also including direction and suggestions for change. It is important to balance positive and negative feedback, not only to make the person feel good, but also to reinforce what has worked well so this might be further replicated and developed.

The provision of feedback is not unidirectional, rather, it is an exchange of information. If we are prepared to give feedback we should also be prepared to receive it, and vice versa, we should be prepared to give feedback if we receive it. Therefore, in any positive professional relationship we need to invite others to provide us with feedback about our performance. In doing so we need to accept others' comments in an attentive and non-defensive manner, encourage them to elaborate and provide details, take the information on board and make changes where appropriate, and finally give recognition to those who have assisted us in our development.

Conclusion

This chapter has been designed to assist in the use of reflective techniques within the professional context. It is through reflective contemplation that we are able to learn from and about practice, and thus further develop our professions. Portfolios are useful tools in both supporting and communicating professional reflection, and therefore are widely used within educational and professional recognition processes. As this chapter has detailed, there are numerous tools that can be used to support and record our professional reflections. It is important to select or develop an approach that meets the needs of a specific situation. Over our careers we will utilise numerous reflective tools and approaches as we develop our practice, plan our careers and contribute to the development of new knowledge. In addition to structuring these activities, these tools also act as artefacts or evidence that can be used when making a claim of competence or further reflecting on our achievements. As the following chapter will elaborate, we need to be cognisant of the quality and generalisability of this evidence, and ensure that our claims and proposals are accurate, robust and well supported.

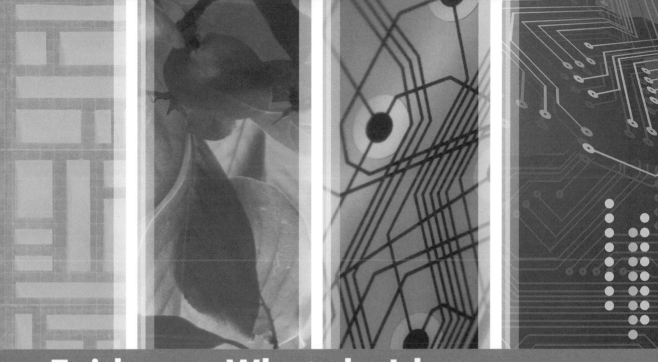

CHAPTER 4

Evidence: What do I have and what do I need?

Introduction

- You need to start collecting items of evidence for your portfolio, but where do you start?
- How do you decide what to collect and how do you judge the quality of the items of evidence?

Chapters 1—3 of this book addressed the 'big picture' to help you understand the overall purpose of a portfolio as a whole. Chapters 4—5 will show you how to put together the various parts of the portfolio so that its aim — namely to produce an account that demonstrates and evaluates progress towards learning and/or professional competence — is achieved. This chapter will introduce the concept of evidence and explore the nature of the quality of evidence and how to use it to support the claims that are made within a portfolio.

A portfolio needs many different types of evidence. Evidence is necessary to support the point your portfolio is attempting to make (Jasper 2006). While

Nursing and Midwifery Portfolios. DOI: 10.1016/B978-0-7295-4078-0.10004-3

single items of evidence may demonstrate particular aspects of practice or learning, the demonstration of professional competence requires a range of information. This information needs to be about your efforts, progress and achievements over time and should be brought together into a coherent argument. It is the combined nature of evidence with a written position or argument of achievement against specified criteria that allows a portfolio to be assessed. In the UK and New Zealand, and previously in some Australian state nursing and midwifery regulatory authorities, portfolios have been assessed as part of the evidence used to make decisions on whether a person's level of professional competence is sufficiently robust for practice. This method is increasingly under scrutiny and, as discussed in Chapter 1, portfolios cannot prove that a portfolio author has a certain level of clinical competency. However, there is a long and well established track record of portfolios having a valuable role to play in demonstrating learning. This learning is certainly evident in the efforts of the person who develops the portfolio and in particular can show development of reflective thinking and writing skills. These skills can communicate what is understood about the professional role and responsibilities through the decisions that are made about what to include in the portfolio. For this reason portfolios can demonstrate to the portfolio author and the portfolio reader a number of components necessary to assessment of competency development.

The following discussion explores a range of issues to consider and potential items of evidence useful in portfolios. It is also important to think about working towards achieving the overall objective of a portfolio. The quality of the accumulated items of evidence will, at least in part, dictate the quality of the overall portfolio. In this way evidence acts as the 'building blocks' that provide substance to an argument of learning and/or professional competence.

Where do I start?

You may be feeling overwhelmed and worried that you have no materials or evidence to begin the task. On the other hand you may have kept comprehensive records throughout your professional studies and employment and be feeling reasonably confident. Even when you need to develop a portfolio from scratch, you may be surprised at the amount of documentation you already possess about your professional learning objectives, outcomes or experiences. You may have various assessment items you produced in undertaking educational or training programmes. If you have been in paid employment or have relevant work experience, or you have engaged in volunteer work you are likely to have some documents that describe the organisation or setting, as well as the role you undertook there. You may even have some feedback about how you performed. Nursing or midwifery students and practitioners accumulate a range of documents about what they do in their studies or in their practice and these can be used to put together an account of professional knowledge, skills and professional performance. These various assessment items and records of work-related activities may include a performance management or clinical assessment report, a case study prepared as part of your studies, a client referral letter, a care plan or a professional reference.

The following discussion will provide examples of the different types of evidence and examine what constitutes a quality item of evidence. It will cover how to collect and produce or generate single evidence items that address a necessary range or variation. It is important to remember that portfolios are always kept for a specific purpose so structure, organisation and content (such as the way ethical issues are addressed) all need to link to this purpose (Jasper 2006). A reassuring reminder at this point is that, no matter what the portfolio purpose, it is always a 'work in progress' that develops and improves over time. It is also important to remember that a portfolio cannot be used to prove or disprove anything. Rather, it is used to support your claim to meet externally assessed requirements.

Whether a portfolio is for assessment of learning outcomes in further or higher education studies or to meet the needs of employment, it is always an illustration or account of individual learning and meanings that are bounded by a range of evidence. The depth and breadth of this evidence is dependent on the original purpose of the portfolio. Although early portfolio versions may not be as comprehensive as you might like, the aim is to include any evidence that allows the portfolio reader (for example your lecturer or manager) to have confidence that learning has occurred and skills are being developed sufficiently at this point in time. It may be useful to start with the notion that the nature of the evidence is more significant than the amount — in short, 'never mind the quality, feel the width'. To get you started in thinking about evidence Figure 4.1 identifies some of the types of evidence that may be included in a portfolio for a practising nurse or midwife (Norman 2008).

What is the purpose of evidence?

The purpose of evidence in a professional portfolio is quite simply to provide some foundation for the claim to some type of achievement. Evidence is used to indicate, show or prove something. As we can see from Figure 4.1, evidence is usually in the form of an object, document, recording or product of some sort. Single items of evidence alone rarely provide enough support to prove or disprove something. The word 'Explanation' has been added to 'Evidence' in the central circle of the figure. This is because the components of the outer circles are objects that only become evidence when they have been considered and discussed in a commentary that provides justification for the inclusion of the individual items in the portfolio and explains how they individually and collectively link to the overall portfolio argument of achievement.

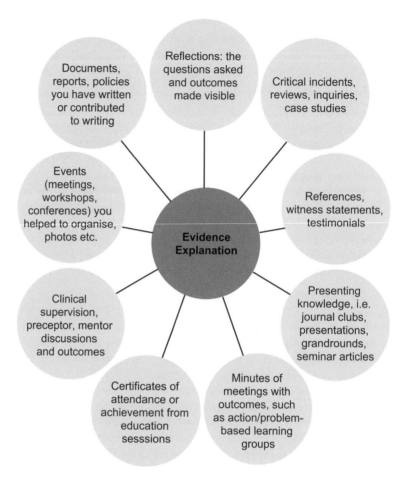

FIGURE 4.1 Types of evidence (modified from Norman 2008, p. 49)

In the same way that, at a trial, lawyers argue for the significance of particular pieces of evidence, so a portfolio needs to argue purposefully why various items can be brought together to create a particular picture. For this reason, careful consideration needs to be given to the reasons for including each item of evidence in a portfolio.

There are now powerful empirical reasons to base healthcare decisions on research evidence (Paley 2006) and health professionals are committed to integrating the latest research evidence into their day-to-day clinical practice in order to deliver the best possible treatment outcomes. The social and professional standards for what the community and our professions accept as quality healthcare now demand an evidence base. Evidence-based practise for health practitioners requires them to give proper consideration to what is the best available evidence and to current practice guidelines, as well as thinking about how these fit with the needs and values of the client and the available clinical expertise (Sackett et al 2000). This definition recognises that research alone is not the only source of evidence and that it may not provide all the information necessary to direct the scope of actions that are undertaken by health professionals in providing safe and appropriate healthcare for their clients.

In addition to research evidence, it is possible to get objective and subjective information from other people, including professional colleagues, co-workers, clients and/or employers, managers or other authorities. Additional information can also come from personal observations, reflections, experi-ences and case studies. Individual client circumstances and the resources that are available in the educational or healthcare context also need to be considered. An effective portfolio will demonstrate individual client and workplace practice as well as your understanding of the impact of the rele-vant healthcare and professional context, including social, political and cultural dimensions. In the case of nurses and midwives, this includes using the professional standards and guidelines and showing how you practise in relation to them.

The use of good quality portfolio evidence shows your awareness and understanding of the required knowledge, skills and attitudes for the level at which you need to practise. It also demonstrates that you are aware of the different characteristics of your learning or practice environments that shape your outcomes and achievements. For example, you may have certificates in breastfeeding support or wound management that will support a claim about current knowledge and skills in these areas. This evidence needs to be supplemented with a description of how you apply this knowledge in your practice. Description of the workplace context is important. As you can imagine, the application of breastfeeding support or wound care knowledge and skills will differ for people in managerial and educational roles. The clinical settings or contexts in which you practice will significantly influence how you use your existing knowledge and skills and how you develop new knowledge and skills. For example, though the principles may be the same, competency in breastfeeding support will be enacted and described quite differently in the context of home-support programmes, delivery suite or midwifery management roles. Similarly, wound care competency will be described differently in the contexts of community nursing, residential aged care or surgical units. In the context of mental health, services may be very different when the nearest specialist is thousands of kilometres away from when the patient and mental health provider are both members of a small community.

Different forms of evidence also serve different purposes: for example, a certificate in breastfeeding support can demonstrate the achievement of a learning plan aim or outcome; a case analysis can demonstrate a level of application and adaptation to client needs; and a client audit can demonstrate planning and analysis skills as specified in an individual role description. Alternatively, one piece of evidence may be used to support more than one claim; for example, certificates for breastfeeding support or wound care can be evidence of achievement of learning as well as evidence of having knowledge and/or skills related to a specific area. A certificate of attendance at an educational session is not in itself evidence of being competent. Levels of competency, particularly for skills, can really only be demonstrated effectively through achievement of assessment or practice outcomes as assessed by a third party.

Discussion so far has outlined how the quality of single items of evidence is important to the formation of your overall portfolio in demonstrating not only reflection on practice but also an informed view on what best practice is and how your practice or learning measures up against this. It is in this sense the broader aim of professional competence.

Summary points: The purpose of evidence

· Evidence in a portfolio establishes a foundation or basis for your argument of achievement (learning outcomes and/or level of competency).

· Evidence will have as many forms as necessary to demonstrate the single or multiple aims of a portfolio and the evidence will also be relevant to each of the various settings or contexts in which learning and practice has or will be required to occur.

· Evidence can stand alone as a collection of single items but needs to be substantiated by consideration of other information and then linked to create an overall claim of achievement.

· It is the quality and range of evidence in a portfolio that allows others to assess and make judgements about the portfolio claims.

What is quality evidence?

Your work in bringing together the best evidence within a portfolio demonstrates a number of things. It shows that you understand and are able to perform some of the necessary skills and practices for your professional role in contemporary healthcare practice. Similarly, it is through using a range of high quality evidence that a portfolio will communicate not only your current competence, but also provide the reader with confidence that the skills demonstrated in the portfolio can be transferred to a range of situations and will be robust; that is, be maintained across time. The very nature of professional practice and the associated notion of individual professional autonomy of practice are premised on the idea that a practitioner will perform at an appropriate level of competency in a range of circumstances, some of which have yet to be encountered (Rafferty et al 2001, Pairman 2005).

Despite the promises of what lifelong learning can bring, we can never be totally confident that a person's abilities and skills will be maintained, or will continue to develop over time or be consistent in different contexts (Smee 2003). For example, the skills acquired through years of experience will differ depending on whether the experience has involved many new challenges or many years of doing the same thing. Even in the one job there are challenges that come with keeping up with new developments, such as the implementation of evidence-based practice.

Evidence becomes quality evidence when it is the most accurate and tangible evidence from a range of primary and secondary sources that is available at that time and over a period of time, and is able to be authenticated, where necessary.

Hence, when deciding if an individual item is of good quality, you need to consider the following:

· What tangible evidence can I use to demonstrate practically this aspect of my practice?
· How best can I demonstrate my performance authentically that shows actual performance?
· Is this current evidence — does it demonstrate my current practice and is it constant with measures of quality contemporary practice?

The following information has been included to assist in addressing these questions.

Tangible in nature

Portfolios may involve written, textual or electronic forms. The very definition of the word 'evidence' is associated with the need for tangible information or data. Tangible evidence is information in a form that another person can view independently in order to judge its quality, that is, the evidence can be authenticated. Hence tangibility is being able to show that evidence is accurate and reliably based on facts or genuine circumstances. A conference presentation is an example that would meet this criterion for those who were in the audience, while some record of the presentation would be needed to make the evidence tangible for those not present at the time. Examples of other types of record or evidence would be a PowerPoint document, video recording or podcast. The best form of evidence of a conference presentation would be the publication of the paper in peer-reviewed conference proceedings; this not only provides a verified and detailed account of the paper, but the peer-review process also provides a form of quality endorsement. Similarly, the written notes or verbal or videotaped recording of a clinical activity also makes the evidence item available and able to be externally assessed although it lacks the inbuilt quality endorsement of a peer-review process. Other examples of tangible evidence of clinical activities include documented health assessments, care plans, referral letters and case presentations. These are objects that can confirm or substantiate what is done in behavioural activities. There will be times when you may need deliberately to produce tangible evidence of some aspect of your professional activity in order to demonstrate this in a portfolio.

A behaviour becomes tangible in practice and is suitable for use in a portfolio where it produces a planned outcome that can be shown in some way. As two examples, wound care and an appropriately sutured episiotomy are visible things that can be observed and evaluated against expected standards. Similarly, improvements in a client's parenting skills or self-management of a chronic condition are measurable outcomes that, at least in part, demonstrate effective practice. Unfortunately, these can be difficult to capture in a portfolio. Photos may assist in some instances and are particularly useful in recording visibly observable changes over time. For instance, wound healing can be photographed over time as a visual record of the success and appropriateness of a prescribed therapy and quality practice. Single items of evidence generally, however, have little meaning when submitted out of context. Depending on the requirements of your portfolio, this example of evidence would need to be supplemented by the inclusion of the context in the form of a more detailed case analysis or clinical report. A contextually-based detailed case analysis, for example, has the potential to transform a range of relatively intangible evidence into documented form, thus allowing others indirectly to observe and evaluate. Where relevant to your area of practice, audit results can also provide a useful form of tangible evidence, particularly when analysed against your role description. Audit results can also demonstrate change when associated with an implementation in which you have been involved, and best practice guidelines or research evidence are other important additions.

Issues of privacy, consent and intent are very important when thinking about evidence. Legal, organisational and professional standards and codes of conduct exist and are designed to protect the interests of persons in hospitals and other healthcare settings. It is reasonable to assume that people in public places may be aware that they may be observed without their consent; however, use of photographs by nurses or midwives may inadvertently breach professional standards if they are obtained and used without appropriate consent. For example, photos of babies and midwives may in some circumstances be represented inappropriately as 'trophies of professional practice'. Privacy, confidentiality and disclosure are important professional considerations and no less so in the development of professional portfolios. Despite photographs being used widely in nursing practice to promote understanding in research, teaching and learning, and as a method of observation, there is limited reporting on how ethical obligations are negotiated (Riley & Manias 2004). It is necessary to get advice from relevant and suitably well-informed colleagues, supervisors, managers or regulatory authority staff if you are planning to use such forms of evidence in your portfolio.

Primary and secondary evidence

The term 'primary evidence' is used in this book to refer to portfolio items or artefacts that are derived directly from practice outcomes such as client care activities and are developed by a practitioner for the portfolio (Jasper 2006, Cooper & Emden 2001). 'Secondary evidence' is information that is provided by a secondary person such as a supervisor, colleague or client and may be used to substantiate claims made within the portfolio. It may also be evidence that already exists and supports the argument being made in the portfolio (Jasper 2006). In reality, there is not a simple or absolute delineation between primary and secondary evidence; rather, evidence ranges across a continuum between information that is directly gained through the provision of client care and information that is completely provided by a secondary source. The relevance here is not so much the definition, but that you will need a combination of both primary and secondary evidence to substantiate your claim of professional competence.

Portfolios, like all other forms of performance assessment, need to be scrutinised for professional and/or academic integrity (Storey & Haigh 2002). It is the requirement of any professional to protect themselves against claims of fraud. The production of fraudulent portfolios is no doubt as widespread as other forms of academic and professional misconduct. One way to communicate that your portfolio is a genuine representation of your performance is to include evidence that is more than just a reflective account, that it is one substantiated by others — that is, secondary evidence. Secondary evidence may be a report of observations of practice with signed assessors' reports of the actual levels achieved, reaccreditation or test results, or a letter of support from a senior colleague substantiating the quality of the services you provide. Similarly, a client may provide a letter of support or you may use an evaluation form to collate feedback about your performance. Some organisations encourage the use of peer evaluation/review processes; at senior levels this may include a wider range of resources such as 360 degree feedback assessments producing useful forms of secondary evidence substantiating your claim of continuing competence.

The quality of the secondary evidence within a portfolio is judged both on what is said and on who is saying it. This is similar to any reference letter; for example, there needs to be congruency between the authority of the author to make specific claims and the claims that are made (Cooper & Emden 2001). In other words, a quality reference needs to be provided by someone who has reason to be familiar with the quality of your work and who has expertise in the area they are commenting upon. Letters from clients are useful to substantiate claims of caring, compassion and, in some situations, currency of knowledge. These need to be mixed with letters of support from a senior colleague, however, to substantiate claims of clinical excellence and technical skill. It is important to align the evidence with the correct performance indicator.

Primary evidence, namely documents and artefacts that are products of your daily practice, need to be judged based on professional standards. As will be detailed in later chapters, when compiling a portfolio it is important to justify the way in which items of evidence demonstrate achievement of specific standards and or competencies as they relate to best practice. Explaining the relationship between an item of evidence and these standards of practice is a vital part of the justification process. It is important, therefore, when collecting primary evidence that consideration is made as to how this might best demonstrate and meet the standards of a profession. For example, do not be tempted to include a case study that had a positive outcome if the evidence and write-up of the situation does not address the necessary course or assessment objective, standard or competency statement. It is important to evaluate the item of evidence for the skills and abilities that you can demonstrate about yourself, including your ability to problem solve and respond to change.

A range of sources

As has been mentioned, evidence used within a portfolio must include a range of items that demonstrate aspects of professional performance. A portfolio for an experienced practitioner may include such items as an employment record linked to position descriptions, letters of support from clients and staff, journal articles or presentations, documents or client instruction sheets developed by the practitioner, and so on. Each item of evidence in the final portfolio is selected to demonstrate aspects of performance. For example, having written a client information handout can demonstrate a range of skills and understandings, such as the ability to write in a clear, concise and appropriate manner, taking into account the literacy skills of the client group; the inclusion of contemporary information; and the desire for client empowerment through the communication of resources and information. However, the development of a client information handout does not demonstrate a range of assessment or clinical skills, and thus there remains a need for diverse sources of information to show evidence of the range of requisite skills to meet the specific professional role.

For most health professionals, case studies are an important means of demonstrating an application of clinical skills. While a single case study may provide a range of portfolio items, such as the client assessment report, care plan, case analysis and more, to use only one case study as a source does not substantiate a claim of flexibility or transferability of competence. Being able to assume some degree of flexibility and transferability of knowledge, skills and attributes is important, even though it is understood that 'skills' and 'traits' commonly accepted as indicative of individuals themselves are often better accounted for by contextual 'states' (Eva 2004). This is why detail about the context of practice and evidence items is important. However, there is no absolute rule or quantifiable measure of the ideal number of case studies as it is the person's professional judgement that needs to be apparent and based on the specific situation. A student or new practitioner may produce an acceptable portfolio using a single case study with other evidence items, such as undergraduate assignments, academic transcripts and clinical assessment reports. An experienced practitioner may have a routine of documenting significant or relevant critical incidents or case studies every 3–6 months, providing them with rich resource of multiple and varied evidence to use.

If you are a student remember to keep notes throughout your clinical or experiential placements of the various things you did and learned each day. Remember also to record not only new things you do but also the areas where you do things with a higher level of competency — such as providing the same care without prompts or remembering to evaluate the effect of your nursing or midwifery intervention — and document accordingly. Such records will be invaluable when writing your portfolio. It is also important to assemble your portfolio as soon as possible after clinical or experiential placements as the longer you wait, the more difficult it becomes to be accurate.

It is also worth thinking beyond your individual performance even though the portfolio is most likely to be used to demonstrate individual achievement. As discussed in Chapter 1, competence is most commonly considered from the individual perspective. However, evidence will exist for most nurses and midwives about inter-professional and team competence. These are the outcomes of a professional group to which you belong and actively contribute. With healthcare becoming increasingly complex we understand that care is now rarely provided in absolute isolation from others. The geographically isolated rural or remote health practitioner usually has some access to technology to enable consultation with and referral to other health professionals. Recognition of patients as the experts of their own health experience also necessitates their central role in decisions about their care.

Education of health professionals about how to work together effectively has been demonstrated in a systematic review to improve some of the ways health professionals take care of patients (Reeves et al 2008). A related idea of 'collective competence' has been studied in a number of settings from aircraft crews to hospital staff (Boreham 2004) and as part of workplace culture (Boreham et al 2000) and work organisation and relationships. Collective competence is understood to be when individuals create shared models of best practice. An example might be where health professionals on a ward or healthcare unit provide competent individual patient care while also knowing collectively what needs to be done for other patients in the ward or unit. This ability would be very familiar to experienced nurses and midwives who work effectively in teams and communicate at regular intervals, as well as covering each other in taking responsibility for patients to ensure patients are safe and quality care is provided while staff take breaks or manage unforeseen events. In this way collective consciousness is more than a combination of individual competencies, with interaction a key feature (Boreham 2004).

Suitability and relevancy

Portfolio items of evidence will be assessed by the reader for their suitability and relevance to the claims of meeting standards of practice or learning objectives. Anxiety about not meeting the required outcomes or standards is a common emotional response to learning or assessment experiences. Most people feel anxious or vulnerable when making information about their work available to others for judgement. However, it is important to note that it is through taking this type of risk that changes in learning and practice occur.

The evaluation of whether an item meets contemporary standards of practice differs according to the nature of the activity. For instance, to have a paper accepted by a peer-reviewed journal or conference is in itself an affirmation that the paper meets a specific standard. With other activities, however, the assessment must be apparent through the demonstrated use of external measures. Many academic items of assessment require that students read widely and demonstrate the integration of a range of external ideas and research findings through academic referencing. Similarly, it is useful to reference the use of professional practice standards when preparing a portfolio item. If preparing a case study, for example, it is recommended that you include references to hospital protocols or the professional literature where appropriate, thus demonstrating familiarity with, and use of, the literature. By aligning your work with practice standards you are able to demonstrate your currency as a practitioner, and therefore the suitability and relevance of your evidence.

Figure 4.2 illustrates further important aspects necessary to reach meaningful conclusions about the quality of your evidence. The three phases in the diagram draw on the work of Pearce (2003) to demonstrate how reflecting on an experience or practice event can be strengthened when considered from different perspectives. Chapter 3 discussed the value of thinking about and reflecting on your actual experiences and professional practice in a particular area. It is also important to make notes and perhaps research further the accepted published science, facts or theory for the particular area or aspect of practice to add another important dimension to your understanding about your practice. This knowledge will help you to assess the quality of your practice and the suitability of the evidence in supporting your portfolio claims. To then review this specific practice against the relevant best available evidence or guidelines adds another layer through which to strengthen your claims.

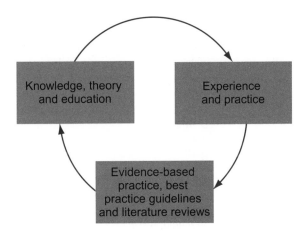

FIGURE 4.2 Making evidence meaningful

As will be explored in Chapter 5, an evidence summary may be useful in highlighting the relationship between items of evidence and contemporary practice. Table 4.1 demonstrates how this may be achieved.

This example shows the selection of a suitable example of evidence for a portfolio demonstrating an understanding of the material outcomes of practice and how these may demonstrate levels of competency. The idea (that a discharge letter is evidence of competency) is supported through a description of the letter contents and assessment of which parts of the letter meet professional requirements of quality. In the example quality standards are deemed to be met by providing accurate information, using an appropriate communication style and highlighting the issues of concern for the care of the patient. This information is then aligned with some of the relevant issues from the current literature on the topic. This example demonstrates knowledge of privacy and confidentiality, duty of care and appropriate standards of communication and skills in informational literacy and application of analysis to practice and evidence-based practice. It could be added to by a commentary or reflective review about the circumstances around this actual practice or the learning that went along with compiling this evidence in this way.

Links between an item of evidence and indicators of quality may not always be apparent to others and may need to be highlighted as part of preparing a quality item of evidence (as in Table 4.1) and through reflective commentary as discussed in Chapter 3 on reflective practice and how this can contribute to portfolios. In cases such as this it would not be unusual to include secondary evidence, such as a supporting letter verifying that the item being discussed is your own work and represents your usual standard.

Although less common in health practitioners' portfolios, photographs, drawings, audiotapes, podcasts and videotapes may also be used as evidence.

TABLE 4.1 Example: Evidence summary

Example evidence item	Details contained within the item	Indicators of quality	Relationship to the literature
Discharge letter to staff of a residential aged care facility	Presented in a professional communicative manner in terms of language use, style and content. The format includes a summary of: · assessment, including risk assessment · relevant care provided during hospitalisation · detailed continued care requirements including medication administration, continence management, bowel status, feeding, hygiene and social needs	· Client and institutional details correct at the time of initial use but deleted for the portfolio submission for reasons of confidentiality · Appropriate introduction summarising reason for letter — thus setting the context for the details provided · Letter designed to focus on potential issues in the rehabilitative phase for this elderly client in order to enhance continuity of care	As identified by Huang & Liang (2005), effective discharge planning and documentation reduces length of hospitalisation and readmissions, and improves activities of daily living. A content analysis of discharge letters for clients hospitalised for post-cardiovascular accident found that many letters omitted sufficient details required for safe transition and continuity of care (Sackley & Pound 2002). Only 37% of the letters had risk assessment detail, while 66% of the letters used broad encompassing terms such as 'needs all care'. The discharge letter referred to in this table adheres to the recommendations of Sackley & Pound (2002)

Evidence for portfolios is usually gathered through what in research terms is understood as unobtrusive methods, that is, information or data collected in a way that does not actively require the participation of others (Liamputtong & Ezzy 2005). The research literature explores the merits and techniques of doing research — that is, getting information and answers to questions — without intruding on people's lives. Regarding the earlier discussion of privacy and confidentiality, it is important to clarify that a range of techniques and sources may be used to generate the best possible portfolio evidence. All information gathering and reporting needs to be conducted in an ethical manner and must not compromise an individual's welfare or rights. Importantly, written consent is required where a portfolio includes the words or images of others. Where consent is not possible the person or persons should not be identifiable.

> ### What is quality evidence?
>
> - Tangible in nature — evidence that is real and can be evaluated
> - Primary and secondary — evidence that already exists and new evidence that needs to be generated for this specific purpose
> - Range of sources — you and the team
> - Evidence that is suitable and relevant
>
> Each item of evidence needs to be tangible in that it provides evidence of some aspect of your practice. There needs to be a range of items — some from primary sources that provide direct evidence of practice, and some from secondary sources that help substantiate the authenticity of your claims. Each item needs to demonstrate quality practice, and thus, where possible, be aligned to evidence-based practice indicators.

Evidence for portfolios

In Chapter 2 we described different approaches to structure a portfolio. Each of the different ways shares some evidence such as employment records and academic transcripts; however, the purpose of the portfolio will determine the required evidence. Table 4.2 describes examples of some of the types of evidence.

As demonstrated in Table 4.2, the type of evidence becomes more complex depending on the purpose and audience for the portfolio. For example, care must be taken in aligning specific items of evidence against the criteria against which the portfolio will be measured, such as the nominated registered nurse or registered midwife competency standard. An understanding of what each of the statements means is clearly very important. In the past state and territory regulatory authorities or organisations, and often employers, provided detailed explanations about the standards, competencies or role descriptions that could form the foundation of a portfolio and related submissions. An example of a guide that was produced to assist with use of these standards was the *Principles for the Assessment of National Competency: Standards for Registered and Enrolled Nurses* (Australian Nursing Council 2002). This was produced before the establishment in 2010 of the single national nursing and midwifery regulatory authority — the Nursing and Midwifery Board of Australia.

Selecting evidence for a portfolio

Ask yourself what existing knowledge, skills and attributes (competencies) or learning outcomes you can demonstrate? If you list a series of competencies of learning outcomes the next question is, What do I have that will allow me

TABLE 4.2 Portfolio evidence examples

Evidence	Examples
A diverse range of documents related to your professional or educational activities and competence. These tend to be records *conveniently* provided by employers or educational institutions rather than deliberately developed by the nurse/midwife for the purpose of a portfolio	Employment record Academic transcripts, awards and certificates Log of continuing educational activities (compulsory and elective) Registration record
Documents developed to demonstrate actions and competence in relation to specific outcomes or objectives. While some documents are *conveniently* available as a consequence of work and educational activities, others are *purposefully* developed to provide evidence of an identified learning outcome	Learning log, reflective/action learning diary Referrals log Educational activities and assignments Justification statement
Documents developed to describe previous actions and competence against predetermined competency criteria — similar to that of a process-orientated portfolio. Often these documents are *purposefully* sought or constructed to address a specific standard	Clinical assessment record Care plan Care intervention summary Referral letters Records of other competency review processes
Documents describe previous actions against predetermined criteria as part of a broader analysis of professional competence. These documents are *purposefully* acquired to address a specific component or competency	Case study Publication (e.g. journal article) Presentation (e.g. conference or seminar)

TABLE 4.3 Example of portfolio structure

1. Personal details
2. Summarising statement
3. Standard 1
    3.1. Statement of justification
    3.2. Evidence summary
4. Standard 2
    4.1. Statement of justification
    4.2. Evidence summary
5. Onwards — continuing through each of the standards that you are using to frame your portfolio
6. Evidence items or appendices
    6.1. Curriculum vitae
    6.2. Academic transcript
    6.3. Position description
    6.4. Case study 1
    6.5. Case study 2, etc.

Search the web page of the Nursing and Midwifery Board of Australia for guides to using the competency standards for nurses and midwives. Are you aware of any interprofessional competency standards that relate to your practice?

Alternatively, resources to assist in understanding criteria may be available through searching the relevant literature. It is recommended that you make yourself familiar with the criteria or standards, carefully checking that you have not misinterpreted or narrowly interpreted any of the statements.

to demonstrate these? For each piece of evidence you think of ask yourself the following questions:

· Is it primary or secondary evidence?
· What is its purpose?
· What does it demonstrate?
· Which learning outcome/objective/assessment criteria or achievement does it relate to?
· Can it be used to support or illustrate more than one point/achievement?
· Which analytical point in the commentary /reflective review does the evidence support?
· How can I reference it in the text?
· Where will I put it in the portfolio?
  (Jasper 2006, p. 163)

To help you identify your existing documents and understand how they help build a portfolio it is important to consider portfolio purpose, outcomes and audience.

List all the potential portfolio documents you already have relating to your professional practice and/or learning as a student. Now consider the following:

1.

    i) What form does the evidence take (e.g. is it something you have written such as a transfer letter, care plan, case study or health information paper or a reflective or commentary piece)?

    ii) What sort of evidence is it (e.g. is it 'convenient' evidence such as provided by an employer or educational institution about compiling a portfolio, or do you have some items that would act as 'purposeful' evidence to demonstrate a process, standard or product.

iii) Think about the quality of the evidence. Using the information provided earlier in this chapter, assess your evidence in relation to the following questions:

- How tangible is the evidence?
- Is it primary or secondary in nature?
- Does all your evidence come from only one or two sources? Are there other sources?
- How suitable and relevant is each document?

2. How does all this evidence come together in addressing the aim of your portfolio?

- What are the strengths and weaknesses?
- Are there any gaps?

At this point you may find it useful to share your information with a fellow student, work colleague or mentor to get their views on the strengths, weaknesses and potential gaps in your evidence.

3. Find and interpret the criteria that are required or might be used to assess this portfolio. It may be professional standards such as those required by a nursing and midwifery regulatory authority, assessment criteria such as those required by an educational provider, or even a position description produced by a potential new employer. Consider the match between the portfolio evidence that you currently have and the type of portfolio you are required to develop or that will best meet your needs. Where are the overlaps and gaps? Is the spread of evidence even across criteria?

In most instances a single item of evidence has the potential to address a range of activities and skills so portfolio structure is important. Chapter 2 discussed portfolio models and structures and the next chapter will address putting a portfolio together; however, a reminder of portfolio structure is useful at this point so the following example of table of contents is provided.

Visualising this format will help you to understand the need to evaluate portfolio items for relevancy to the specific standards that make up the framework you are using to structure your portfolio. It is not unusual to accumulate a range of portfolio evidence items that address a single competency statement or component of performance and yet have insufficient items for other areas. For instance, nurses and midwives may have access to client assessment and referral documents prepared as part of their daily activities, and are therefore able to demonstrate competence associated with documentation skills. For most nurses and midwives, however, unless they have been presenting to their peers or undertaking further studies, the experience of compiling evidence into a case study is not common. Therefore, where portfolios are introduced as a requirement of professional regulation, it is important that this is done in association with supportive staff development and changes to performance management processes. In doing so it is important that professional development activities are designed to provide tangible evidence that can be contributed to portfolios.

You have a range of evidence, and what next?

This chapter was designed to help you identify what constitutes quality evidence. This is assessed by having a range of items of evidence with each item being substantial and related to some aspect of your practice. Items need to be partly from primary sources that provide direct evidence of practice, and some from secondary sources that help substantiate the authenticity of your claims. Each item needs to demonstrate quality practice, and thus, where possible, be aligned to evidence-based practice indicators. As will be explored in Chapter 5, collecting a range of quality evidence items, though a vital part of compiling a quality portfolio, is only the beginning. Your next step will be to put together your evidence and match it against each of the performance indicators/competency statements. This will high-light any gaps in evidence you have and may require that you generate or put together additional evidence. The concept of quality evidence is central to this process, for it is only through the compilation of quality evidence that you will be able to achieve a quality portfolio.

The following activity has been designed to help you reflect on items of evidence and consider how the quality of these might be assessed and enhanced. Further, this will assist you to understand, and hence explain, the relationship between individual items of evidence and the claim of compe-tence being made.

Activity

Select a significant item of evidence, and using the diagram below, in:

> Box A — record the competency or learning area you would attribute this evidence to.
> Box B — describe the item of evidence according to the practice activity of learning experience it demonstrates.
> Box C — list the factual information that informed your actions for the relevant item of evidence.
> Box D — provided a list of all the relevant best-practice evidence and/ or professional guidelines related to this topic area/practice.

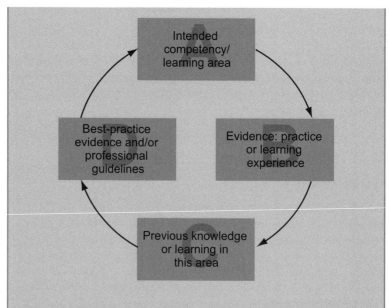

Intended
competency/
learning area

Evidence: practice
or learning
experience

Previous knowledge
or learning in
this area

Best-practice
evidence and/or
professional
guidelines

Having completed each of the boxes, reflect on the quality and relevance of the item of evidence. The following questions will assist with this.

· Is there alignment between the evidence and the competency/ learning area?
· Does the evidence reflect sound knowledge and best practice principles?
· Is this a suitable item of evidence — or could I improve upon this (for example, would a commentary be useful in demonstrating further learning and practice development).

The above activity could be used for each item of evidence. Figure 4.3 (a blank version of Figure 4.1) 'Types of Evidence' illustrates, how this activity would relate to the multiple examples of evidence required for a portfolio. This would be a considerable amount of work and all of it may not always be necessary, but it is a useful exercise in identifying the foundations of current and best practice.

This chapter has examined the nature and purpose of quality evidence, plus how to recognize it, produce it and enhance it. Understanding how evidence informs and supports a portfolio is essential in producing a quality product, be it a claim of achievement or providing direction for learning and professional growth. Similarly, recognising the quality of individual items of evidence is necessary both in selecting those that are relevant and enhancing existing items. Having achieved this, you are now in a position to commence assembling your portfolio, where these items of evidence will be used to substantiate your claims of achievement and inform further learning.

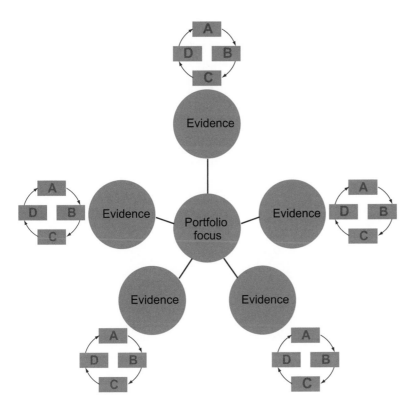

FIGURE 4.3 Reflecting on the quality of your evidence

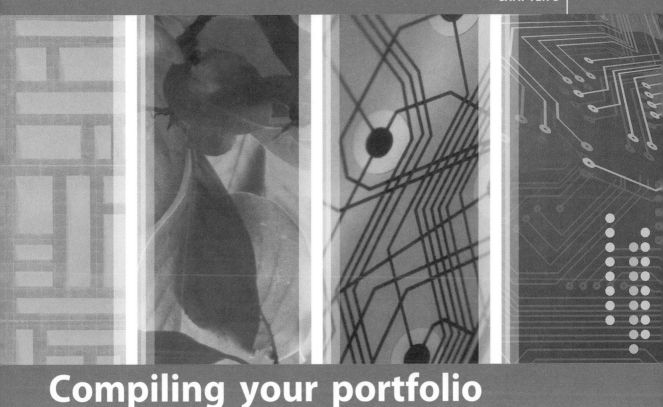

CHAPTER 5

Compiling your portfolio

Introduction

· You understand the aims of a portfolio in developing reflective thinking, communicating learning and achievement in studies for entry to nursing and midwifery practice, and for recording practice and continuing professional development. You also understand the need for and features of quality evidence. Now you need to consider the evidence you already have and start developing your portfolio.

· Alternatively you have a portfolio developed for a specific course and now want to expand, reorganise or restructure it for a different purpose.

This chapter will guide you in creating a portfolio, with activities to assist you included throughout the chapter. If you have not already started we suggest you write answers or make notes in a Word file or notebook as you read through the chapter so that you can build sections of your portfolio as you look at the descriptions and explanations.

The production of a quality portfolio is undertaken progressively, over time, as you consider a series of interrelating steps. These steps are as follows:

1. Selecting the appropriate portfolio framework. In some cases this may involve accessing a prescribed framework or template such as from an employer.

Nursing and Midwifery Portfolios. DOI: 10.1016/B978-0-7295-4078-0.10005-5

2. Consideration of your learning plan and collection of information or evidence.
3. Identifying gaps and generating new evidence to address these. This may include writing commentary that justifies the portfolio parts.
4. Reviewing and organising the contents of your portfolio to ensure the materials correspond to the overall portfolio requirements.

Your knowledge and experience will influence how you follow the suggested pathway in building a portfolio. For instance, you may be compiling an e-portfolio and have a solid understanding of the framework and concepts you want, or need to use. In this instance you will move straight to reviewing existing evidence. If, however, you are new to portfolios, it may be a better use of your time to consider how you will frame the portfolio in the first instance before moving through the other steps.

Deciding on and designing a portfolio framework

A portfolio's strength lies in organisational clarity, cross-referencing, quality evidence and quality analysis (Emden et al 2003). In order to achieve this it is imperative to develop a plan early in the development process (Cooper & Emden 2001). Therefore, having gained some understanding of portfolios, it will be useful for you to develop a schema of what your portfolio will look like, thus helping you to frame your 'project' and give you an indication of the sort of information you will need to compile and develop. As previously indicated, some professional organisations have provided ready-made portfolio formats, either in text form (e.g. Nursing Council of New Zealand 2008) or via an e-portfolio interface (e.g. Royal College of Nursing Australia 2006). To assist midwives in the compulsory competency review process for re-certification, the New Zealand College of Midwives produces and makes available for purchase structured portfolio frameworks.

The purpose of your portfolio will inform what will be the most appropriate framework for your portfolio. If your portfolio is for an application for your first job as a nurse or midwife then use of the relevant national standards will be important. If the portfolio is for performance review by your employer then close attention to the requirements of your job description and the nursing and midwifery continuing professional development standards will be important. Development of a portfolio (or a section to be included in a portfolio) as an assessment item in a course should include a clear outline of the learning outcomes that need to be achieved and demonstrated. Knowing these learning outcomes will help inform the portfolio structure.

Regardless of which of these are the drivers for your portfolio development, we recommend designing your table of contents first. This will help clarify the professional and personal images that you are aiming to communicate to the reader of your portfolio. In effect, a table of contents is a plan; it will appear at the front of your portfolio as a list of or index to the various components of the portfolio. All headings will clearly relate to the purpose of your portfolio. In Chapter 3 we introduced the use of a table of contents as a way of visualising an entire portfolio. The following framework is an extension of this and includes an explanation of each of the portfolio components. Having reviewed this information, you will be ready to commence the activities included to assist you in designing your own.

Suggested framework for a portfolio

Personal details

This first section is the same as would be included in a résumé. It may be omitted in an educational or learning portfolio. It requires a summary of your personal details such as your

· name
· contact details — phone, email, postal address
· professional registration details
· qualifications and education
· summary of employment
· current position description
· professional memberships
· names, titles and contact details of referees.

You are likely also to choose to address broader skills, attributes, experiences or activities such as required by an educational or employing institution. These must be relevant to the purpose of a portfolio and should not overly duplicate material included elsewhere. The Nursing Council of New Zealand and Nursing and Midwifery Board of Australia both provide a number of examples in various documents about competency and continuing professional development. The Midwifery Council of New Zealand is very specific in its requirements for a portfolio from midwives and seeks evidence of competence to practise as well as the application of learning to practise (Midwifery Council of New Zealand 2008). This is specified in point values as evidence of compulsory education, evidence of continuing education and professional development activities as well as application of learning to midwifery practice.

A more generic example of additional items would include

· personal career goals
· scope of practice statement
· a summary of recent continuing professional development plans and activities (including points accrued if relevant)
· publications and/or presentations and research activities
· relevant volunteer work, or related skills and qualifications such as a driver's licence, first-aid certificate, etc.
· police check, immunisation and health records.

Summary statement of arguments or claims

The objective of an introductory statement is to give the reader a sense of the overall purpose, claims and plan of the portfolio, thus preparing them to understand the intention of the portfolio before focusing on specific details. In effect you will be describing the portfolio model, and hence the content of this statement will differ between process-orientated, standards-based and product-orientated portfolios. The main purpose of this statement is to address

· the purpose of the portfolio
· how the purpose is to be achieved
· if appropriate, the relationship between the portfolio, your current and expected scope of practice, career, educational and learning goals.

An example of how you might start your summary statement for a portfolio framed around the Australian competency standards for the registered nurse would be as follows:

> *This portfolio has been designed to provide documentary evidence of my competence as a registered nurse as part of my regulatory requirements with the Nursing and Midwifery Board of Australia (NMBA) and through my scope of practice as a registered nurse in the area of acute care. In order to achieve this, the registered nurse competency domains have been used as the main framework with examples of evidence used to demonstrate both my current performance and developing skills in the area of surgical nursing.*

The above summary statement becomes a declaration of your competence to practise within the specified nursing or midwifery scope of practice.

Alternatively, a summary statement for a course-related portfolio might read as follows:

> *This portfolio has been designed to provide documentary evidence of my learning as part of the course objectives and assessment requirements for … course/assessment. The course objectives/assessment requirements have been used as a portfolio framework with examples of evidence included to demonstrate … (development and outcomes).*

While you are likely to need to change your summary statement as your portfolio progresses, it is useful to develop a draft statement early because this will help you to clarify the overall purpose of the exercise and start you on the way. Like the table of contents, the summary statement will provide a useful reference point for you to refer back to as you build the portfolio and select, alter and even omit materials in the final version. For example, if you find yourself struggling with sections or aspects of the portfolio, refer back to this first statement and ask yourself:

· What are my knowledge skills or abilities for which I need evidence?
· How is this material relevant to the overall aim of the portfolio?
· Which competency or aspect of learning does it address?

- Do I want to include examples about thinking, learning, operation or practice skills or strategies?
- What makes this a quality example?

The answers to these questions will help you clarify which materials to include and what to keep on file for future reference.

Standard or competency domain 1

Statement of justification for why arguments of claims can be accepted
A statement of justification is an explanation of how competence or learning has been demonstrated by detailing how each of the items within the evidence summary table (Table 5.1) is a demonstration of this specific competency statement. In addition to explaining the link between the items of evidence and the competency statement or learning objective, the statement of justification details how these items are a demonstration of contemporary practice or effective learning, and hence show a level of quality achievement.

Evidence summary table
An evidence summary table provides a tabulated display of which items are included as evidence to support your argument of competence, where these items can be located and, if appropriate, which specific component of the competency, domain or learning objective the evidence addresses. In the first instance use this as a working document to list the items you think appropriate for each subcategory, with a brief description of why they have been included in each category. As you progress with your portfolio, this reasoning can help develop your statement of justification. Once the statement of justification is complete you can delete your written notes and replace them with numerical equivalence that will link them to the specific subcategory within the broader competency statement. Note that each item

TABLE 5.1 Example: Evidence summary table

Evidence title	Appendix	Specific subcategory

Case study Elderly male with type 2 diabetes	Appendix 2	Write notes here — include an explanation of the client assessment undertaken and a completed assessment form. Specify how you will be relating your evidence to competency statements 5.1 and 5.2 from the ANMC *Provision and coordination of care* domain (ANMC 2005b).
		5.1 Demonstrates a structured approach namely
		   · a head-to-toe physical assessment and health history using an assessment form.
		5.2 Demonstrates the use of a range of data-gathering techniques, namely
		   · interview
		   · observation
		   · physical assessment
		   · medical practitioner's letter and other secondary information sources.

of evidence may address more than one subcategory. Table 5.1 provides an example of how you might start your evidence summary table that would inform your statement of justification.

The statement of justification and evidence summary table should be repeated for each of the required competencies/standards.

Appendices

The purpose of appendices is to provide supplements referred to in the main text, thus supporting the veracity of the claims being made. The benefit of certain reference items being included as appendices is that they are maintained in full, rather than being presented as excerpts within the main text. The appendices are a combination of the items of evidence you have compiled for the purpose of the portfolio together with other institutional policy documents that are sufficiently integral to the portfolio purpose to warrant being included. In the case of e-portfolios, the appendices are unlikely to be at the end of the webfolio, rather embedded as links throughout. As previously discussed in Chapter 2, these linked items can be in range of digital forms, including links to external sources such as institutional documents or conference proceedings.

One group of portfolio appendices will need to be the items of evidence that you have compiled. With a few exceptions, the size and complexity of the items of evidence you will be compiling make it inappropriate to imbed these as whole items within the portfolio because the flow or argument within the portfolio would be disrupted. An alternative to this is to imbed smaller components of evidence, although this then diminishes the integrity of the evidence itself. For example, a complex item of evidence such as a case study is much more informative when available as a complete entity, rather than when it is provided as small portions and extracts included in the broader argument. Further, these items are likely to demonstrate a range of skills and be applicable to a range of competency subcategories. Thus a case study can be referred to in the main text under several competency statements, while the quality associated with the whole can be maintained by its inclusion as an appendix. Remember that it is important for the relevance of an appendix item to be clearly articulated in the main text.

Examples of items of evidence that may be included are as follows:

- learning objectives and associated achievements such as academic transcripts or completed case studies, concept maps and other educational assignments or presentations
- an employment summary
- continuing professional development attendance details as specified in the relevant regulatory authority documents such as the Nursing and Midwifery Board of Australia Continuing Professional Development Standard
- competency assessments, test results/certificates of attainment for completion of clinical skills including cardiopulmonary resuscitation,

TABLE 5.2 Suggested portfolio framework

Personal details		
Summary statement	· Purpose of the portfolio · How the purpose is to be achieved · Relationship between this portfolio, your current and expected scope of practice, career, educational and learning goals	
Standard or competency domain 1	e.g. ANMC Professional Practice domain: 1. Practices in accordance with legislation affecting nursing practice and healthcare (Australian Nursing and Midwifery Council 2006)	Specific subcategory details
Statement of justification for why arguments/claims can be accepted		
Evidence summary	Title of evidence	Appendix number
Standard or competency domain 2, etc.	e.g. ANMC Professional Practice domain: 2. Practices within a professional and ethical nursing framework (Australian Nursing and Midwifery Council 2006) and so forth …	
Statement of justification		
Evidence summary	Title of evidence	Appendix number
Appendices	Items of evidence such as · curriculum vitae · academic transcripts · position description · case study 1 · case study 2, etc.	Specific subcategory details

medication calculation emergency procedures or supervision and assessment skills, etc.

· referee reports and testimonials
· professional practice/clinical assessment documentation
· a reflective journal, which may include a diary outlining a typical working week
· care plans, case notes or other work-related documents
· presentations, publications and/or photographic records
· research proposals or quality initiatives in policy development.

The second group of portfolio appendices refers to supporting institutional documents that help frame your practice. These documents might include

· professional competency standards
· codes of ethics/conduct
· organisational policies
· other institutional documents such as role descriptions.

A cautionary note here: These institutional documents should only be included if they are highly relevant and not readily accessed by the reader. Many of these documents are available online and a reference to the online source may be adequate, or in the case of an e-portfolio embedded as a link.

The headings that have been suggested in this section have been compiled within Table 5.2 to provide an understanding of how a product-orientated portfolio might look.

Once you have reviewed Table 5.2 you will be ready to start completing your own table. The template provided in Table 5.3 is intended for your personal use. Look back at the activities from the previous chapter and review the evidence examples you identified whether your portfolio is related to entry to registration studies or continuing professional development for the clinician. You will be asked to undertake a series of activities using this table. You may wish to photocopy the pages or write directly into this book. Fill in the sections as suggested.

Resources

Both the Australia and New Zealand nursing and midwifery regulatory authorities recognise ongoing learning as part of their re-certification processes. You can access online the relevant standards, information and guidelines or suggested templates provided on websites by the professional and regulatory authorities (Nursing and Midwifery Board of Australian 2010, Nursing Council of New Zealand 2008, Midwifery Council of New Zealand 2008).

As an example, the requirements of the NMBA Continuing Professional Development Registration Standard for nurses and midwives specifies the following requirements

1. Nurses on the nurses' register will participate in at least 20 hours of continuing nursing professional development per year.

2. Midwives on the midwives' register will participate in at least 20 hours of continuing midwifery professional development per year.

3. Registered nurses and midwives who hold scheduled medicines endorsements or endorsements as nurse or midwife practitioners under the National Law must complete at least 10 hours per year in education related to their endorsement.

4. One hour of active learning will equal one hour of CPD. It is the nurse or midwife's responsibility to calculate how many hours of active learning have taken place. If CPD activities are relevant to both nursing and midwifery professions, those activities may be counted in each portfolio of professional development.

5. The CPD must be relevant to the nurse or midwife's context of practice.

6. Nurses and midwives must keep written documentation of CPD that demonstrates evidence of completion of a minimum of 20 hours of CPD per year.

7. Documentation of self-directed CPD must include dates, a brief description of the outcomes, and the number of hours spent in each activity. All evidence should be verified. It must demonstrate that the nurse or midwife has:

   a) identified and prioritised their learning needs, based on an evaluation of their practice against the relevant competency or professional practice standards

   b) developed a learning plan based on identified learning needs

   c) participated in effective learning activities relevant to their learning needs

   d) reflected on the value of the learning activities or the effect that participation will have on their practice.

8. Participation in mandatory skills acquisition may be counted as CPD.

9. The Board's role includes monitoring the competence of nurses and midwives; the Board will therefore conduct an annual audit of a number of nurses and midwives registered in Australia (Nursing and Midwifery Board of Australia 2010).

Collecting information or evidence

It is now time to compile the pre-existing evidence for your portfolio. Your most recent educational and practice-based experiences are likely to influence the type of evidence that you have readily at your disposal.

As discussed in Chapter 3, a range of types of evidence is needed to substantiate the complex claim of competence. In particular, you will need a variety of evidence that addresses the breadth of your practice, including

TABLE 5.3 Template

Personal details	Decide what should be included in the summary of your personal details, such as (delete and add as relevant)
	• name
	• contact details – phone, email, postal address
	• registration details
	• qualifications/education
	• employment summary
	• current position description
	• professional membership
	• referees' names and contact details
	• personal career goals
	• scope of practice statement
	• learning plan plus summary of recent continuing professional development plans and activities and points accrued if relevant)
	• publications and/or presentations
	• research activities
	• relevant volunteer work and related skills and qualifications such as a drivers licence, first-aid certificate, etc.
	• police check, immunisation and health records
Summary statement	Summarise the purpose of the portfolio and give a brief overview of how you plan to achieve this purpose:
Standard or competency domain 1	Transcribe the relevant standard/competency domain here:
Statement of justification	
Evidence summary	Title of evidence Appendix number Specific subcategory

Standard or competency domain 2	Transcribe the relevant standard/competency domain statement here:		
Statement of justification			
Evidence summary	Title of evidence	Appendix number	Specific subcategory
Standard or competency domain 3	Transcribe the relevant standard/competency domain statement here:		
Statement of justification			
Evidence summary	Title of evidence	Appendix number	Specific subcategory
Standard or competency domain 4	Transcribe the relevant standard/competency domain statement here:		
Statement of justification			
Evidence summary	Title of evidence	Appendix number	Specific subcategory
Appendices			

items from both primary and secondary sources. To recap, primary evidence refers to artefacts or texts that pre-exist as a consequence of what you have done in work, study or in practice as part of your professional activities. Examples of primary evidence are care plans, discharge letters, clinical notes, photographs and assignments. Secondary evidence refers to information that is provided by someone such as a supervisor, colleague or client and may be used to substantiate claims made within the portfolio. You will need to make a judgement about how recent an item needs to be for currency; this depends on the nature of the item and your practice. For example, a case study that deals with an unusual situation but demonstrates a specific legal aspect to your practice may remain current for 5–8 years.

Table 5.4 will help you to think about the range of information you might consider when compiling your portfolio. As you will note, the items of evidence have been categorised against generic competency statements or standards that are suggested to have relevance to most health professionals. These have been developed specifically for inclusion here as a demonstration. When compiling your evidence it is recommended that you use the competency domains or standards that are specific to your role.

From the lists in Table 5.4, including items you may have added yourself, select those items that are of sufficient quality and relevance to be included in your portfolio. As explained in Chapter 3, quality evidence needs to be current and represent contemporary standards of practice.

Next you should title your pre-existing evidence and include the titles in the relevant evidence summary tables, adding notes on how each item of evidence meets the standard or competency. It is also useful at this point to list each of the items within the appendices; you may or may not wish to use numbers for the appendices at this stage as the order or appearance may change. The process of labelling and transposing information within your portfolio is simplified, as discussed in Chapter 2, if you are using an e-portfolio.

Identifying omissions and generating new evidence

Now that you have entered your items of evidence within the evidence summary tables you will be able to identify which competency categories are well supported with a range of quality evidence and where omissions exist. You will now have a basis on which to consider what evidence you will need to generate to support your wider claim of competence.

How do you know how much evidence is enough? There is no single answer to this question because it depends on a range of variables and your personal circumstances. The amount of evidence might be relatively small if, for instance, as a student you are required to submit a prescribed list of portfolio

TABLE 5.4 Details of portfolio evidence

General categories relevant to practice standards	Examples of evidence to support claims. Which of these types of evidence do you already have or what needs to be done to get them?
Practice: in accordance with relevant · legislation · ethics · standards/codes of conduct and practice · scope of practice/decision-making frameworks	· Explanatory statement/table clarifying your understanding of the links between your role description, scope of practice, reporting management framework and other legislative and policy responsibilities · Client case study — needs to refer to relevant legislation, regulatory guidelines and/or institutional policies · Client case study, workplace exemplar and/or supportive letter that demonstrates your applied understanding and preparedness to act in an ethical, culturally competent and professionally responsible manner · Example of case note entries that demonstrate knowledge and skills of regulatory documentation guidelines · Letter from insurance company or employer website address detailing current insurance cover* · Copy of annual practising certificate · Educational qualifications or professional membership for practice according to profession legislation/code of practice · Other:
Communication: demonstrates relevant skills · verbal and written · team work and interdisciplinary collaboration · referral mechanisms	· Letters or other professional artefacts that demonstrate written skills · Case study demonstrating verbal communication skills and professional networking · Position description detailing reporting and referral mechanisms · Example of referral/discharge letter that demonstrates quality referral and written skills · References/testimonials provided by clients or professional colleagues detailing your communication skills · Attendance at professional development activities related to developing and using communication skills · Details of professional presentations given · Other:
Assessment and planning: · for individual clients and/or groups in a range of situations relevant to the context of	· Position descriptions detailing client assessment responsibilities · Client case studies detailing assessment and plan of care, including

(Continued)

TABLE 5.4 Details of portfolio evidence—*cont'd*

General categories relevant to practice standards	Examples of evidence to support claims. Which of these types of evidence do you already have or what needs to be done to get them?
employment or practice (e.g. emergency, multicultural perspective)	<ul><li>direct client assessment (interview and physical examination)</li><li>the use of supplementary information sources in assessing the client's needs</li><li>plan of care that represents both the client's needs and contemporary practice</li></ul><ul><li>Completed assessment documentation demonstrating understanding and application of a theoretical framework/structured approach</li><li>References/testimonials provided by clients or professional colleagues that include comments about your assessment and planning skills</li><li>Attendance at, and participation in, relevant professional development activities</li><li>Other:</li></ul>
Delivery of care:<ul><li>planning and implementation of care</li><li>supervising and managing others</li><li>collaborating with an interdisciplinary healthcare team</li></ul>	<ul><li>Position description and scope of practice statement detailing client management responsibilities</li><li>Exemplars detailing plan of client care you have implemented for a range of clients/client groups</li><li>Artefacts such as photos detailing client progress</li><li>Performance review documentation detailing the quality of care you have provided while employed</li><li>Client and/or peer testimonials detailing the quality of care</li><li>An incident analysis that details your skills and performance in the delegation of care</li><li>Descriptions of health education activities undertaken</li><li>Other:</li></ul>
Evaluation of practice:<ul><li>client outcomes and appropriate modification of care</li><li>institutional processes</li></ul>	<ul><li>Client case study detailing the evaluation of care undertaken</li><li>Audit report or process related to an aspect of your practice</li><li>Supervisor's report or a performance review process commenting on your self-evaluation and client evaluation skills</li><li>Reflective journal demonstrating a high level of self-reflection and professional critique</li><li>Exemplar detailing activities contributing to review and development of institutional policies/guidelines</li><li>Other:</li></ul>

TABLE 5.4 Details of portfolio evidence—*cont'd*

General categories relevant to practice standards	Examples of evidence to support claims. Which of these types of evidence do you already have or what needs to be done to get them?

Contribution to the profession:
· participation and contribution to research activities
· implementation of evidence-based practice
· professional development of self and others
	· Membership of and contribution to
	  · professional organisations
	  · workplace committees
	  · community groups·
	Research articles or other publications·
	Details of presentations delivered·
	Literature review·
	Case study demonstrating use of recognised contemporary practice and evidence-based practice principles·
	Documents detailing educational support provided to others·
	Performance review documentation that includes comment on your skills and activities in this area·
	List of professional development activities undertaken·
	Other:

Personal development	The previous sections have addressed what you do in your professional practice. The focus of this section would be in demonstrating how you practice, how you develop your practice, and how you learn from experience. It would include reflective analysis of your own behaviour in the following ways
	  · explorations of particular patient encounters
	  · objective reviews of your role in critical incidents or working groups such as journal clubs
	  · analysis of how you developed your learning plan
	  · reflections on annual performance appraisal

*Insurance cover is a regulatory requirement for some health professionals including nurses and midwives.

items as a course assessment, with the aim of the assessment being to demonstrate your applied understanding of that aspect of portfolio compilation and justification (Campbell et al 2000). In this case the restricted numbers of evidence items requested would be sufficient. However, if you are compiling a portfolio to substantiate your learning outcomes or argument or claim of competence to perform within a specific role, something much more substantial is required. The full scope of the relevant standards or criteria would need to be addressed within your portfolio.

The remainder of this chapter has been written for those planning to compile a comprehensive portfolio to support a claim of professional competence. Nevertheless, it will still have relevance to those developing a learning portfolio and, therefore, even if you do not wish to undertake this exercise in its entirety, we recommend that you review the process since the principles involved will inform your understanding of portfolio construction.

At this stage it is important to re-familiarise yourself with the requirements of the organisation to which you will be submitting your portfolio. This may mean closely reviewing your key regulatory documents such as competency state-ments, scope of practice documents, decision-making frameworks, portfolio assessment processes and/or schemas and employer requirements. It is during this process that you need to consider what these organisations value and hence what you need to communicate clearly through your portfolio. If, for example, your regulatory organisation provides a checklist of requirements then it is obviously important that you follow this in detail. In most cases, however, this will be a broad guide only, with no prescriptive list detailing the type and scope of all evidence requirements for your portfolio. This is perhaps because both the nature of practice and individual professionals vary so much, and as quickly as such a guideline might be developed it would be superseded by changes in practice. Also, the requirement for such detail might arguably be suggested to be contrary to the principles of professionalism.

As discussed in Chapter 1, the ability to assess and articulate our own competence and scope of practice is central to self-regulation and current notions of professionalism. Nurses and midwives need to possess the level of competence for both day-to-day practice and for the future, to remain part of the flexible and responsive health workforce. Given this, competency stan-dards and similar regulatory guidelines generally provide relatively broad descriptions of practice requirements, thus allowing the range of variations that sit within nursing and midwifery practice.

So how should you proceed with the broad nature of the competency standards provided? Revisit the activity at the end of Chapter 1 and review your list of standards and/or competencies in light of your expected scope of professional practice. Next review your job documentation or position description. Highlight those sections you consider to be essential aspects to your role and indicative of your scope of practice. In other words: What are the important skills you use every day? What are the skills that you may use less regularly but are nevertheless essential to your role (e.g. in emergency situations associated with your role)? What are some background skills that reflect your understanding of your risk management, regulatory and professional frameworks? While a complete portfolio needs to include evidence that addresses all standards, the specifics need to reflect your own particular situation and knowledge.

Over the last decade there have been a growing number of guidelines on the scope of practice and decision-making frameworks developed by Australian health and nursing and midwifery regulatory authorities. To assist in engaging critically with these documents, read the *National Framework for the Development of Decision-Making Tools for Nursing and Midwifery Practice* (ANMC 2007). This document provides a set of principles as a foundation for the development and evaluation of decision-making tools and provides templates for decision-making tools for nursing (registered and enrolled nurses 1) and one for midwifery. In your searches of nursing and midwifery regulatory authority websites you may have noted other decision-making or scope of practice publications. They are worth reading and offer frameworks suitable to examine a particular clinical incident. For example, the nursing decision-making guide is available on the NMBA website. Take a case study or critical incident from your practice and consider the framework questions about client needs, scope of practice and standards, the context or setting and who should provide the care or intervention. Working through a case or incident from your practice may also help you identify a learning plan to develop the skill set to enable you to provide or improve the care in similar circumstances in the future.

Moving on with building your portfolio, we suggest you review the contents of Table 5.4 and reflect on the areas not well represented by the evidence you already have. Once you have compiled a list of the additional evidence you will need to complete your portfolio — where to next?

First, you may find that you do already have an item that will cover the area identified but had not previously seen the connection or relationship. It may be a useful exercise to see in how many places in your portfolio a particular piece of evidence can be used.

Second, consider whether you need to increase the range of evidence in your portfolio. It is also important that you select a form of evidence that best demonstrates the knowledge, skills and attitudes associated with the competency skill you are seeking to highlight or support. For example, a table listing the regulation that frames your practice and how this might be applied in practice is a useful way of demonstrating your associated knowledge, but not necessarily your attitudes as applied in the practice setting. An accompanying reference letter from your supervisor detailing your diligence in following through with your legal obligations, however, will provide the supportive evidence required. This may mean that you will need to enlist the assistance of others in compiling your portfolio evidence.

Third, you may have identified that some aspects of your practice or learning are incomplete and you need to undertake additional training or extend aspects of your current role before you can generate the evidence required.

A fourth idea might be to share your 'work in progress' with a friend or colleague who is also a health practitioner in order to brainstorm new ideas. Alternatively you may approach a supervisor, mentor or lecturer to get more structured feedback on strengths, limitations and gaps to assist you in moving forward to completion. You might review the nature and types of evidence to see if stronger evidence can be obtained through different forms, such as statements written by others, publications or references to your contribution elsewhere, such as in organisational, unit or committee reports.

Other questions you might use to evaluate your portfolio include:

· Are the central claims and justification statements clear and consistent throughout the document?
· Does the portfolio have both breadth and depth of evidence?
· Is there balance in the focus, sources and types of evidence and information?
· Is the portfolio discussion and evidence focused on persons (individuals and groups), actions, knowledge, skills, attitudes and values?
· What is the balance in the portfolio between creative, descriptive, factual and detailed information?
· Are there unexamined assumptions or values that need to be challenged, better explained or removed?
· What style of language has been used? Is there any jargon or vague terminology? Is it objective or subjective?
· Are terms used consistently? For example, have you described providing care to patients, clients or healthcare consumers? Which term best communicates your intentions? Have you used any specific terms of language prescribed by the regulatory authority or employing organisation?
· Are all sections useful in building the arguments and adding support or is there padding in some sections where nothing new is being added?
· Are any statements distracting from your main purpose of the portfolio?
· Do a reality check. Does this portfolio show the best of what you have done in either your practice or learning?
· Does the portfolio hold together as a supported account of your achievements?
· Does it hold together literally in terms of style, presentation and binding? Or, if you have developed an online portfolio, are the pages well constructed with active links?

There are not necessarily right or wrong answers to these questions. The best answers will come through careful reading of your portfolio and consideration of how well it incorporates any required criteria or standards in meeting the portfolio purpose.

Conclusion

This chapter has examined how to identify, create, collect and organise evidence in a professional portfolio. Considerable detail has been provided on how to structure your portfolio, including generating your argument, producing summary and justification statements, and embedding the evidence to achieve the strongest support for your claims for learning. If you have followed the suggested steps carefully it is likely that your last task will be simple. The final product needs to be reviewed to ensure that the arguments of achievement or statements of claim are supported and justified by the organisation and evidence within the portfolio. Chapter 6 will provide more detail and guidelines about assessing and evaluating portfolios.

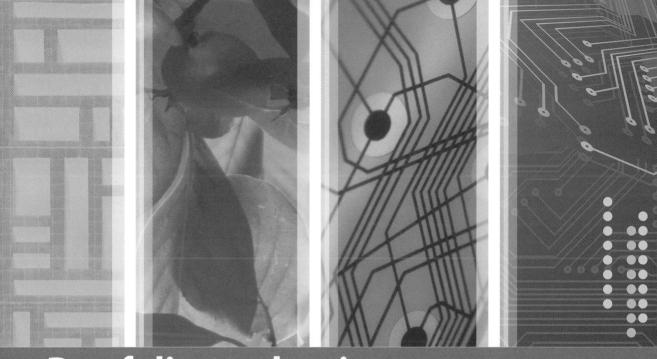

CHAPTER 6

Portfolio evaluation and assessment

Introduction

- · You are a health professional or student developing your portfolio and want to understand better the perspective of the assessor who might be evaluating your product.
- · You are a lecturer considering introducing portfolios as a student assessment task.
- · You are a member of an appointment or promotion committee seeking guidelines on how to assess the value of individual portfolios.

The focus of this chapter is on assessment of professional portfolios. Portfolios are commonly used in education as assessment items to support learning and provide a measure of student/applicant achievement. Equally, anyone reviewing a portfolio as part of a promotion application or the like is undertaking an assessment. As this chapter details, portfolios are assessed for different reasons and the reason will influence the appropriateness of assessment approaches. For instance, if the purpose of the assessment is to

Nursing and Midwifery Portfolios. DOI: 10.1016/B978-0-7295-4078-0.10006-7
Copyright © 2011, Elsevier Australia.

provide direction for future learning, as it is with a learning portfolio, then the feedback mechanisms and details need to be focused towards this end. Alternatively, if the purpose of the assessment is to provide a summative judgement about performance or achievement, then the associated achievement criteria should be very apparent in the assessment rubric/ feedback sheet. In addition to the traditional notions of assessment, portfolios may also be used as part of an institution's audit system as a cluster of data to evaluate the institution's success in supporting student and staff performance outcomes. In this way, information generated through assessment of individual portfolios can inform the development and review of relevant policies, guidelines and criteria, including the need for staff development. To take advantage of these opportunities, however, and ensure that assessment practices do achieve the intended outcomes of supporting learning and/or ascertaining the achievement of performance criteria, quality assessment design is an imperative.

While this chapter has been written for current and future assessors of portfolios, people compiling their own portfolio will also benefit from understanding the perspective of the assessor when preparing their portfolio or reviewing the assessment feedback. The chapter includes an overview of portfolio assessment and evaluation, as this understanding is necessary to inform the design of quality assessment processes that stimulate learning and quality reporting mechanisms. Various exemplars and activities have also been included to assist the reader in applying these principles to practice.

Portfolio approaches and the impact on assessment

In Chapter 2, it was proposed that there are two major portfolio approaches, namely the 'process-orientated' or learning portfolio and the 'product-orientated' or achievement portfolio (Barrett 2009). The process-orientated approach is a formative, educative and process-driven approach that highlights the processes of recording, mapping and moving towards personalised professional or practice development goals. The second 'product'- or 'achievement'-orientated portfolio approach is about demonstrating the achievement of a standard for the purposes of accreditation, promotion or gaining recognition of an accomplishment of some kind. There is of course some overlap between these two approaches, in that most learning or process portfolios do require achievement outcomes, and most product or achievement portfolios need to make an argument for demonstrated continued progression in relevant learning. Even so, assessment processes do need to attend to the major purpose of a portfolio in order to inform and support the student/staff member in achieving and being rewarded for the intended outcome. As will be discussed here, the appropriateness of an assessment approach will vary as a consequence of the differing purposes of these two portfolio approaches.

In the case of an educational or learning portfolio, assessment is undertaken to support continuous improvement using feedback that is designed to engage and support the student/staff in their further learning (Ewell 2008). As a consequence, the assessment needs to reward successful use of reflection, critical evaluation, soundness of planning and achievement/ critique of personalised learning outcomes. As will be elaborated upon later in this chapter, assessment rubrics and other forms of feedback frameworks are useful in making these sorts of achievement components apparent to the learner and providing a focus for feedback. Similarly in-text and comment-based feedback within a learning portfolio should be learning-focused and hence provide explanations of learning processes, direction to resources and provide relevant inspirational examples. This form of feedback is usually a cyclical, ongoing process where advice and feedback are given over time with the intention of continued growth and development.

Assessment of a product/achievement portfolio has accountability as its central tenet, whereby the assessor is responsible for ensuring a set of predetermined standards are maintained (Ewell 2008). As a consequence the assessment framework needs to provide a clear reference to the performance standards being assessed, and the criteria being used to make the final judgement. Feedback may include direction for continued improvement, but, importantly, needs to clarify the basis of the final decision regarding success or otherwise of attaining the required outcome. Both those being assessed and those auditing the assessors need to be able to see how a judgement, grade or other decision was arrived at. Prescribed requirements, such as those written by regulatory authorities or professional organisations, need to be very evident within the assessment criteria and feedback provided.

As we have previously indicated, many portfolios require description and evidence of both processes and outcomes and so this dichotomous comparison between 'process' and 'product' portfolios may not always be apparent in practice. However, it is a useful basis initially to examine your portfolio and consider the assessment approach that might be most appropriate. Table 6.1 highlights the two extremes of portfolio style and the different ways that purpose, structure and assessment may be approached in each of these.

Summary points

- The central tenet in the assessment of educational or learning portfolios is to support and direct continuous improvement, and in doing so to support and reward the processes of self-assessment reflection, planning and implementation.
- The central tenet in the assessment of product/achievement portfolios is accountability of achievement, and in doing so to support and reward the framing of a claim that is substantiated with sufficient quality evidence to ensure a set of predetermined standards are maintained.

TABLE 6.1 Two professional portfolio approaches

	Process-orientated	Product-orientated
Portfolio purpose	*Development/continuous improvement* Promotes student and/or professional nurse or midwife self-assessment and development across specified areas of knowledge, skills and attitudes. May include what has occurred in the building of the portfolio, including reflective aspects of self-assessment, planning and progress. Records and reflections of interactions related to the stages, journey or development of student/staff learning and progress is a strong element.	*Demonstration of achievement* Makes a particular and definitive argument or case for achievement, usually for certification or re-certification of licence to practise, for promotion or Recognition of Prior Learning (RPL). The focus is on an end-product that demonstrates the best possible argument, case or presentation of the necessary level of performance or achievement against a set standard.
Portfolio structure and organisation including evidence types and use	*Personalised structure, chronological substructure* Structure can vary, with portfolio authors potentially choosing an approach and the materials for inclusion that best supports their learning. Because the purpose of this portfolio is to demonstrate learning over time, a chronological substructure is commonly used.	*Prescribed thematic structure* The portfolio is organised according to a clear prescribed structure that may be criteria, standards and/or outcomes, as prescribed by the institution 'applied' to. Materials may be limited to those stipulated by the portfolio assessor as necessary and the author may not be required to interpret the evidence.
Portfolio assessment	*Integrated or holistic* The purpose of this assessment is to engage the author for the purposes of continuous improvement. Formative or ongoing assessment is common and may or may not result in a final/formal assessment judgement/grade. For grading purposes, the complete collection of materials or record of development is assessed against the author's claims of self-understanding and professional development. Assessment criteria are focused on the author's ability to: assess a situation, critically reflect, plan, effect change and evaluate outcomes. In addition to providing recognition of quality learning processed, feedback should also include direction and resources for learning.	*Methodological or systematic* The purpose of the assessment is to ensure a set standard is met, particularly in the case of accreditation, promotion and RPL. The assessor is accountable to the institution to ensure compliance with these prescribed standards, and therefore will draw on these and broader notions of 'in the public/institution's interest' in making their decision. Therefore issues of patient and public safety must be clearly attended to. The portfolio is assessed systematically according to criteria such as educational, statutory, professional or organisational standards or outcomes. Feedback needs to include clarifying and justifying the assessment decisions.

Portfolio assessment and evaluation

While the terms assessment and evaluation are commonly used interchangeably, particularly in the professional practice context, their meaning in the professional/educational setting is not necessarily the same. In this context evaluation generally describes the broader process of institutional appraisal and feedback, whereas assessment pertains to the learning/performance outcomes of the individual. A rather simplistic definition would be that a student or staff member's work is assessed, while an organisation's performance is evaluated. The relevance of this definition within this text is that the assessment of individual portfolios (belonging to students, applicants or staff members) can be useful in informing the institution's evaluation process. While this chapter will mostly address the assessment process in education, it is important to consider how portfolio assessment results, or portfolios more generally, could provide useful evaluation data to inform healthcare and educational intuitions' evaluation of student and staff performance outcomes and needs. If portfolios, or the data related to the assessment of portfolios, were to be used in this manner, it would be appropriate that information and possibly consent be sought from the students/staff during the submission process.

Why assess?

While there is a range of reasons why educational providers, employing organisations and regulators might use assessment processes, these can generally be reduced to two broad and potentially overlapping categories, namely to

·   direct and stimulate student/staff/applicant learning, including self understanding
·   regulate/accredit/communicate professional/educational standards (Boud & Solomon 2001).

As previously discussed, both of these purposes influence the way in which assessments are designed and what criteria are used to pass judgement on the outcomes. While it is essential for the assessor to understand this if they are to provide high quality, rigorous and consistent assessment processes, it is also useful for the learner/applicant to understand the perspective of the assessor. The following activity is designed to support both the assessor and the person being assessed to understand the range of learning or performance outcomes that might be developed and assessed via a portfolio.

Activity: Intended portfolio outcomes

Table 6.2 has been constructed for you to complete. The aim is for you to consider a range of intended learning outcomes for both learning/process portfolios and achievement/product portfolios. To achieve this you will need to list the different portfolios and portfolio activities that you are aware of, and then:

- consider which of these have a learning process or achievement product as the purpose
- list each portfolio title within the appropriate column
- under each portfolio title, list the intended outcomes (learning or achievement).

To assist, examples have been included in the table.

TABLE 6.2 Intended portfolio outcomes

Purpose: Demonstrating learning process	Purpose: Demonstrating product achievement
Example: Title: Annual continuous professional development (CPD) for continued registration portfolio Learning processes and outcomes: - identifying personal learning needs - developing a learning plan - maintaining records about the plan implementation including reflecting upon the impact of the various learning experience. Title 2: ……..	Example: Title: Promotion application portfolio Performance outcomes: - leadership - clinical expertise - change agent - high level communication skills - ongoing/lifelong learning Title 2: ……..

Assessing to direct and stimulate learning

It has been long understood that assessment is a major influence on what and how students learn (Boud & Falchikov 2006, Biggs & Tang 2007). From a learner's perspective, the requirements of assessments clarify what is 'truly' valued and rewarded by the assessor/institution (André 2002). In doing so, assessment provides the incentive and direction for student learning. The assessment activity not only informs the learner about the content that needs to be learnt, but also fosters skills and attitudes about learning (André 2002). For instance, process skills such as teamwork, communication and critical thinking can be developed and refined almost accidently while developing an assessment product such as a poster presentation, essay or staff development presentation. Quality assessment activities that reward the learner for using a solid learning process and meeting quality outcomes have the potential to instil positive values about learning and the application of knowledge to enhance practice.

It is important to note that assessment tasks can also stimulate less desirable learning outcomes. Poorly framed assessments have the potential to encourage and reward superficial learning through the use of rote learning and surface learning (Quinn & Hughes 2007). For example, students can mistakenly use practice exams and quizzes as their primary source of learning, rather than developing a deep understanding of the materials and then using the practice assessment to self-assess. Similarly, poorly designed assessment items that support the direct replication of lecture content may initially be appealing to the learner, but do little to support application and critiquing skills. Sadly learners who have been rewarded by superficial learning can come to resent assessment items that require these higher level learning skills. Hence the impact of poorly designed assessment and feedback practices has potential to extend beyond a missed learning opportunity, and create a lasting negativity towards learning and change in general. Ideally, quality assessment items are designed not only to support deep, applied and effective learning, but also provide transparency, resources and formative feedback that supports learners in understanding their broader achievements (Boud & Falchikov 2006). The objective is for professionals to be habitual deep, applied and motivated and discerning learners.

Portfolios are commonly used in education as a learning activities and assessment items (Jasper & Fulton 2005, Bryne et al 2009, Green et al 2009, Karlowicz 2010). Equally, anyone reviewing a portfolio as part of a promotion application or the like is assessing a portfolio. As has been identified, complex activities such as assembling a portfolio, especially if laden with new skills and terminology, have the potential to misdirect and obscure student/staff learning and further stimulate attitudes of anti-intellectualism among participants (Scholes et al 2004). In their eagerness to teach new skills and understandings, educators (including those in staff development) often 'frontload' learning experiences with terminology and theory frameworks, rather than engaging the students/staff in activities that would support progressive skill acquisition. Many of us will have experienced this in our early exposure to nursing/midwifery theory, research methods and critical thinking. Unless done well, the teaching and assessment of these often conceptual topics can result in students failing to meet the deep and applied learning outcomes intended. It is important that the designers of assessment items think about this and design assessments in association with educational support that will enable the intended learning outcomes.

Portfolio development has been identified as influential in developing student and staff attitudes to self-determination, evidence-based practice, professional accountability, application of theory to practice and responsiveness to change (Pearce 2003, Stuart 2004, Australian Learning and Teaching Council 2008, Australian Flexible Learning Framework 2009). These outcomes, however, are only achieved if integrated into a broader curriculum or institutional system that supports progressive student or staff development in a range of associated knowledge, skills and attitudes. It is important to remind ourselves that a single assessment item rarely has a significant and ongoing influence on learning and performance outcomes. Rather, learning is progressive, cumulative and responsive to the broader cultural environment, such that in addition to providing quality assessment support it is also important to have a learning culture that supports openness and risk taking and rewards genuine achievements.

Following on from this sentiment, the large and complex nature of compiling a portfolio means that this exercise is best undertaken progressively over time, with a tolerance of developing ideas and achievements. The challenge for the educator is to design a programme of study and assessment that will support the requisite skills and understandings without distorting student or staff learning such that irrelevant or superficial learning takes precedence over genuine and effective outcomes. Learning can be distorted, for example, if portfolio users are overly distracted by the technology or terminology used to explain aspects of the portfolio, and this becomes the learning at the expense of the intended learning outcomes including reflective learning or understanding of personal competence. Similar issues occur, for example, when the technical/formatting aspects of referencing are taught in a manner that distracts students from understanding the need to evaluate sourced information for relevance and quality. Of concern is that if portfolio users do not see the value of compiling a portfolio, or of framing their arguments, there is a risk that the exercise will be interpreted as rhetorical and burdensome, and potentially reinforce anti-intellectual and anti-management attitudes.

As identified above, it is important to be cognisant of both the intended and unintended learning outcomes that may result from any assessment item. Designing quality assessment experiences requires that students are provided with learning supports and opportunities that will enhance their understanding and skills in achieving this intended student learning. When introducing students to the use and value of portfolios, for example, one recommended approach is to use scaffolded assessment items, such that students accumulate items of evidence and/or reflective learning activities in preparation for undertaking the complex task of assembling a more complete portfolio (Andre & van Eck 2010). The objective of this exercise is to have students undertake smaller assessment activities to introduce the concepts of reflective learning and self-evaluation, while also accumulating performance outcomes/artefacts, in a more controlled fashion. These principles can then be extended when students are undertaking a larger portfolio activity later in their programme of study, for instance when required to deliver a portfolio for a position application using genuine artefacts.

Early in an individual's professional development, detailed directions for portfolio development may help guide their learning activities; this may be reduced later in the programme when the objective is for students or applicants to demonstrate initiative and self-direction. For this reason, for example, direction given to nurse practitioner applicants in developing their portfolios may be deliberately broad, because the ability to evaluate and assimilate a range of materials in order to develop and substantiate an original argument would be considered integral to the performance requirements at that level. If this is the objective, then in addition to informing the applicants of what is expected, the assessment process needs to reward the achievement of this outcome. In some instances the reward will be a higher grade, in other cases, such as for the nurse practitioner applicant, the demonstration of higher-level analysis is a requirement for professional entry.

Assessing for accreditation or employment purposes

Ensuring that students or applicants meet a required standard is a central tenet of any educational or employment assessment. The 'gate-keeping' role of regulators, educationalists and employers is central to their particular purpose. Assessment for competence, either at entry level or as part of continuing registration, must also provide a degree of predictability that the successful student or applicant will maintain safe practice in the future (also referred to as predictive validity) (Quinn & Hughes 2007). Similarly, students, staff members and applicants need to receive recognition of their achievements and the quality of their performance because this will motivate future learning and development.

To meet the requirement of predictive validity identified above, a portfolio must be made up of evidence of sufficient quality. This means that the evidence items within the portfolio need to

· demonstrate currency and contemporary practice
· contain a reflective or evaluative component
· attend to the standard/competency identified
· be validated by others
· be accumulated over time and in a range of circumstances.

Further, the items of evidence need to form a cohesive whole that supports the claim/argument of competence. In order to ensure that this is achieved, concepts of quality and wholeness must be reflected in assessment instructions and then again in the grading/assessment criteria.

In short, the need to direct, encourage and reward specific outcomes will shape the way in which you design and communicate the assessment process. The questions you may wish to ask yourself are:

· What do you want to assess (the content of the portfolio, namely items of evidence and/or the demonstrated process of compiling and justifying a portfolio)?
· How should the assessment objectives and process be communicated to the applicant/student?
· How will assessment rigour, validity and reliability be met?

Your answers to these questions will influence the assessment process you develop. Further sections of this chapter will further assist you in this process.

Summary points

· Portfolios may be used as assessment items to direct learning and provide recognition of achievement.

· In addition to providing an assessment opportunity, staff and student portfolios contain potentially useful evaluation data to gauge the institution's success in supporting student and staff performance outcomes.

· While assessment is a major driver of learning, importantly this may include quality (deep, applied and intended) learning, or unintended learning such as surface learning and attitudinal development that impairs future learning.

· Assessing for accreditation requires 'predictive validity' to be met in order to be assured of continued performance in altered contexts. Assessments should therefore support and reward well framed and appropriate claims that are adequately supported by quality, diverse and verifiable evidence that has been accumulated over time.

What is to be assessed?

As with any assessment process, it is important to clarify from the outset what is being assessed (assessment/learning objectives) and how it is to be evaluated (assessment/feedback schema). It is important to pay considerable attention to this in the assessment design stages. Portfolios can be used to support learning and assess any number of outcomes including demonstrating self-determination through:

· reflecting upon and framing a claim of competence/achievement
· substantiating a claim using a range of quality evidence
· assessing personal learning needs
· developing relevant learning and career plans
· evaluating the success of achievements.

Importantly, 'producing a portfolio' is not in itself a learning objective; rather the portfolio is a tool to achieve a more specific objective, for example those listed above.

For the purposes of the remainder of this section, it will be assumed that the broad objectives of what is to be assessed have been set. In some cases these will be learning objectives accompanied by detailed assessment instructions. In other instances such as promotion applications or position applications, the applicant will need to interpret these through reflecting on the task required.

Whatever the situation, it is important to consider the overall 'intent' of the assessment/portfolio requirement throughout the assembly and assessment process, because this will help you to clarify the priorities that should be explicit in both the portfolio and the assessment feedback framework.

As the following information will detail, the learning objectives and broader intended learning outcomes will inform the appropriateness of grading structures and assessment feedback schemas.

Awarding grades

The following discussion pertains to the assessment processes associated with awarding grades, namely incremental merit-based grades (for example 'pass' through to 'distinction') or criterion-referenced grades (for example pass/fail). Where it is intended that assessment outcomes need to reward a range of levels of performance, it is generally appropriate that grades extend beyond unsatisfactory and satisfactory, to include higher levels of merit such as credit and distinction. This form of graded assessment originates from the concept of 'norm-referenced assessment'. In an early approach to norm-referenced assessment, grades were distributed according to a predetermined distribution across the candidate population, based on the normal distribution curve, also referred to as a 'bell shaped curve' (Quinn & Hughes 2007). In this traditional form, grades were attributed according to the students' comparative rankings (Frisbie & Waltman 2006). The contemporary use of norm-referenced assessment generally no longer requires this. Rather, grades are awarded according to a set of predetermined criteria whereby, for example, if all students performed at the required level, they could all receive a distinction grade. Hence the more accurate term now is 'incremental graded assessment', rather than norm-referenced assessment.

Criterion-referenced assessment, often referred to as 'non-graded pass/fail', is an alternative form of assessment grading. This approach is often used in instances where a range of higher-level achievements cannot be reliably or easily assessed, and so an outcome of 'achieved' or 'not achieved' is most appropriate. This is not to say that the assessment is less rigorous; on the contrary, pass marks may be as high as 100%, because an underlying premise of criterion-referenced assessment is that the pass criteria reflect the minimum standard of practice required. Criterion-referenced assessment is most commonly used for assessment of skills where it is either irrelevant or difficult to set criteria that would assist in reliably determining high or advanced levels of skills (Frisbie & Waltman 2006). For example, criterion-referenced assessment is usually used for assessing technical skills where the requirement is that the applicant meets a minimum level of performance, such as proficiency in performing cardiopulmonary resuscitation. Similarly criterion-referenced assessment is often used when evaluating portfolios for regulation and promotion purposes, because it is both irrelevant and difficult to ascertain qualitative differences beyond the required 'acceptable level of performance'.

There are instances where the two forms of grading are combined. For example, a fail grade might be awarded if proficiency in a specific criterion, such as referencing, is not achieved, irrespective of other achievements in the assessment. Having met this criterion, however, the work is then graded using an incremental graded system. These 'assessment hurdles' should be used sparingly, and in instances where proficiency has been structured into a programme of study (Best & Best 2009).

As discussed, the desired learning outcomes will inform the assessment approach to be used. From an educational perspective, incremental graded assessment is important in communicating and rewarding the merit of students' work; however, there are times when criterion-referenced assessment is more appropriate. Many regulators will use non-graded pass/fail criteria in a manner that demonstrates to their stakeholders acceptable and unacceptable standards of practice. In the educational setting, however, non-graded assessment outcomes are problematic because the merit of the student's performance is not communicated to the student and through their academic record. Academic records and associated calculations such as grade point averages are used often as the initial screening process for employers and educational institutions. It is therefore important that grades awarded to students reflect the range of their achievements, and are not limited to learning outcomes that are traditionally accepted as 'easier to grade'. This is the very argument for the grading of clinical practice in undergraduate programmes, for example (André 2000).

The alternative when assessing large and complex items such as portfolios is for educators to consider specific learning outcomes. For example, it might be appropriate in the first instance to assess individual portfolio items, with a particular focus on the concept of quality evidence. In later stages of the course, students may be required to submit a more complete portfolio with the assessment grade being awarded to the quality of the rationale and argument. By using this approach the student is rewarded for specific learning outcomes, while at the same time compiling a larger work.

Having identified whether incremental graded assessment or criterion-referenced assessment is to be used, it is necessary to develop a marking or assessment schema. How this is achieved will depend on the assessment approach being used. For both approaches, however, it is imperative that the assessment criteria are designed to evaluate the learning/assessment objectives identified and that they are clearly understood by those involved. The concepts that have been identified as the 'criteria of quality' will also inform the grading details of the schema. For instance, earlier in this book we referred to indicators of quality evidence as items that are current, relate to contemporary practice and demonstrate the performance outcomes relevant to the competency/standard in question. It is important to have the indicators of quality inform the design of a scoring schema or rubric, so that the pre-established criteria against which the student's or applicant's work is to be evaluated are clearly detailed.

A scoring rubric, compared with a checklist, is probably the most common form of scoring instrument used for evaluating a performance task (Mertler 2001). The format of a rubric can vary but typically includes a rating scale against which either the components of the product or the product as a whole are judged. Table 6.3 demonstrates an analytic rubric whereby the rating scale is detailed against a list of the components of the larger product. In Table 6.3, the activity of a client assessment has been used to demonstrate the concept of rubrics.

Table 6.3 has been included for demonstration purposes only and is not a complete analytic rubric. The first column details the components of the assessment task that ideally would have been taught in class or be available in some educational form. The assignment components listed may be assigned a percentage as part of awarding an overall grade (Mertler 2001).

The top row of Table 6.3 details the scoring criteria. As shown in this example, the range of grades are not necessarily a consequence of the frequency of behaviours, rather, qualitative increments are added to the aggregation of content. The qualitative increments detailed in Table 6.3 have been informed by the work of Biggs and Tang (2007). A range of parameters may be used depending on the qualities that are relevant for the activities, including descriptors of 'dependence to independence' (Bondy 1983) and 'novice to expert' (Benner 1984, Spence 2004).

The cell content of the table provides detailed descriptors of how the broader grading criteria may be applied to the specified assessment component. As you will note from this example, even at this level of detail some interpretation is required. It is important that this interpretation is part of the moderation processes that will be outlined in this chapter about validity and reliability of assessment.

Table 6.4 is an example of a criterion-referenced assessment approach, which might be more appropriate within the regulatory or staff development context. Table 6.4 illustrates the use of binary response (e.g. yes/no) associated with a criterion-referenced assessment approach. It is important to note that such an approach is not necessarily easier to implement. Both incremental graded assessment and criterion-referenced assessment approaches require substantial support mechanisms to assist applicants and assessors to understand and apply the assessment process.

Student/applicant feedback

As demonstrated in Tables 6.3 and 6.4, it is possible to provide a significant amount of information to students, staff and applicants about the assessment process. It is now expected that if using quality teaching practices, assessment processes and information should be provided to students/

TABLE 6.3 Example: Scoring rubric

Assessment item: Develop and utilise an appropriate tool to be used to evaluate your teaching

Assessment components	Advanced	Proficient	Functional	Developing: minimal pass	Unsatisfactory
	The learner is able to demonstrate extension beyond proficient to include insightful questioning and development of hypotheses and theories	*The learner offers an integrated understanding of all essential aspects, such that the whole has coherent structure and meaning*	*The learner focuses on the relevant area and works appropriately with all the essential aspects. The learner provides correct materials with discrete and separate pieces of information*	*The learner focuses on the relevant area but requires direction in some non-essential aspects*	*The learner is engaged in the task, but is distracted or misled by irrelevant aspects*
Quality of discussion including presentation of ideas, concepts in a logical and systematic manner. Demonstration of understanding of assessment and evaluation through the application and evaluation of concepts and theories to own practice.	Proficient criteria plus – Consistent links made between course content and application to the context of this assignment. Early levels of analysis and critique of course materials applied in the context of this assignment. Extended quality literature used effectively to support emerging arguments. Original and creative thinking demonstrated.	Functional criteria plus – Extended comprehension and application of course materials to the context of the teaching session described. Theories and concepts explained well with regular links between course content and application to the context of this assignment. Some extension beyond materials supplied within course content.	Coherent and logical basic comprehension of course materials and consistent beginning levels of application. Components include: Overview of evaluation and assessment approaches that were considered. Sound justification of approach selected, including relevance to the context of the sessions described.* Summarises evaluation results accurately and comprehensively.* Details how future practices have been informed by findings. *Essential criteria – all must be completed appropriately*	Predominantly sound understanding of course materials with occasional confusing or incorrect components. Application of course materials present with some limitations. Requires direction in one or more of essential 'functional' components	Minimal to poor levels of knowledge and understanding of assessment and evaluation. Consistent errors in minor aspects of knowledge – OR Failure to demonstrate understanding of significant aspect of course content including: Evaluation and assessment approaches used. Summary of results. Impact upon future practices.

Demonstration of the use of critical thinking to gather, evaluate and deploy relevant information to assist in problem-solving and synthesis.	Evidence of appropriate and effective use of contemporary literature. Evidence of robust critique.	Materials beyond recommended readings used effectively. Evaluation and assessment outcomes evaluated at depth with a beginning level of critique of either the literature or the approach selected.	Adequate range of readings used. Concepts identified in the literature well integrated and applied within the body of this work. Occasional linking statements demonstrating application and relevance to assignment purpose.	Minimal range of readings. Opportunities for critical and analytical discussion missed on more than two occasions but overall a sound level of knowledge and understanding demonstrated.	Inadequate range of readings used.
Deployment of quality literature to develop and understanding, argument and application.	Proficient criteria plus – Wide range of credible and relevant literature that exceeds course materials, with material comprehensively and appropriately integrated into assignment discussion.	Functional criteria plus – Use of quality multiple in-text citations and/or integration of concepts from the literature. More than the stipulated range of quality sources used.	Paraphrasing of authors' ideas to indicate points of view. Few direct quotations. Stipulated range of relevant sources as per course materials.	Mostly paraphrasing of authors' ideas to indicate points of view; some direct quotations. Stipulated range of relevant sources used as in the course materials. Some sources less credible.	Stipulated range of relevant sources as in the CIB, not used. Some sources less credible. Numerous direct quotes with occasional paraphrasing. Some statements not referenced.

TABLE 6.4 Example: Criterion-referenced assessment checklist (possible)

Nurse Practitioner Competency Framework Standard 1:

Dynamic practice that incorporates application of high-level knowledge and skills in extended practice across stable, unpredictable and complex situations (Australian Nursing and Midwifery Council 2005a)

Competency 1.1: Conducts advanced, comprehensive and holistic health assessment relevant to a specialist field of practice (Australian Nursing and Midwifery Council 2008a)

Is there a coherent and informative structure, namely:

· Is there a clear and comprehensive *claim of competence* that sets the scene and clarifies the range and relevance of health assessment skills for the specific clinical specialty and client population? Yes/No

· Is there a comprehensive list of *items of evidence*? Yes/No

· Is there a *justification statement* that explains the relevance of each of the items of evidence that links to the claim of competence? Yes/No

CLAIM OF COMPETENCE

Are you satisfied with the quality of the statement/claim of competence, namely does it clearly:

· state the competency area being claimed (namely health assessment)

· state the scope of skills relevant to the specific specialty, including those needed in stable, unpredictable and complex situations

· demonstrate relevance to the client population?

Yes/No

Comments:

ITEMS OF EVIDENCE

Item of evidence	Maintains client confidentiality	Verifiable	Reflects contemporary practice standard	Relevant to claim	Included in justification statements
	Yes/No Comment:	Yes/No Comment:	Yes/No Comment:	Yes/No Comment:	Yes/No Comment:
	Yes/No Comment:	Yes/No Comment:	Yes/No Comment:	Yes/No Comment:	Yes/No Comment:
	Yes/No Comment:	Yes/No Comment:	Yes/No Comment:	Yes/No Comment:	Yes/No Comment:

JUSTIFICATION STATEMENT

Does the justification statement and the evidence listed with in this address the following performance indicators

Performance indicator 1	Yes/No			Explain your judgement:
Performance indicator 2	Yes/No			Explain your judgement:

FINAL DECISION

Based on the above information, has this applicant met the requirements of this competency? Yes/No
Comments:

applicants well in advance, with many educational organisations providing grading schemas as part of the assignment instructions. Complex tasks such as the assembling of a portfolio require additional support; students and applicants gain considerable assistance from discussions with those who will be evaluating their portfolios (Scholes et al 2004). The inclusion of a formative assessment process, whereby feedback and direction are provided part way through an assessment activity, is particularly important for large and complex assessment activities such as portfolio submissions (Jasper & Fulton 2005). These feedback comments may be embedded within the text of the assessment activity and/or presented as a written/verbal summary.

The nature and extent of feedback comments are generally dependent upon the time and resources available, plus also the purpose of the assessment. In formative assessment situations, where students and applicants may use feedback to improve upon the assessment activity, the feedback needs to provide both direction and incentive to do this. The inclusion of both broad and detailed direction, plus links to resources and explanations using exemplars to demonstrate the applications of principles, are useful strategies to achieve this. Within summative assessment situations, in addition to formative feedback, it is also important that clarification be provided about the basis of the final decision or grade. Statements that demonstrate the alignment between performance aspects of the portfolio and the assessment grading criteria are useful to help the applicant/student understand how and why the final grade/decision was awarded. It is just as important for the student/applicant to understand why they were successful as it is for them to understand what else could be achieved.

In both summative and formative assessment situations, it is important the feedback reflects the intent of the assessment, and therefore includes comment about the holistic direction of the assignment, rather than overly emphasising specific components such as editorial changes.

Validity and reliability of assessment

Ensuring both validity (assessing what is intended and not something else) and reliability (consistency within the assessment process and between assessors) is clearly of concern when assessing portfolios (Roberts & O'Rouke 2002, McMullan et al 2003, Webb et al 2003, Spence 2004). As has been discussed earlier, poorly designed assessment activities, or lack of learning resources to support an outcome, can mean that assessment items distract from, rather than support, student/staff learning. This lack of validity has been observed when technical processes associated with e-portfolios, for example, override the intended learning. Similarly assessment outcomes should be consistent, such that the process is fair and reliable, no matter who the assessor is.

As a consequence of the need for reliability and protection against plagiarism, the assessment process may include further verification such as referees reports or a presentation/'portfolio defence' requirement. A 'portfolio defence' is where an applicant provides a presentation exemplifying aspects of their portfolio and is available to respond to questions. This was a common requirement for nurse practitioner application processes, for example, prior to the introduction and availability of accredited programmes of study. In some respects, a job interview is a form of portfolio defence also.

To a large extent, assessment validity and reliability can be maintained through the design and formulation of a clear grading schema. However, the reliability of an assessment schema can only be maintained if accompanied by a rigorous assessment moderation process (Webb et al 2003). It is recommended that a moderation process include a range of the following:

· external review of teaching materials and assessments by a credible outsider in order to benchmark and validate the rigour and other standards of assessment
· internal moderation involving a range of review mechanisms including
    · opportunities for markers to work as a group to define, clarify and refine the assessment requirements and marking schema
    · blind double-marking of a group of assignments/submissions early in the marking process further to clarify the marking schema and justify the grades/results awarded
    · review markers' grading distributions both midway and at the completion of marking groups of assignments (i.e. if numbers of assignments/submissions are sufficient the frequency of the range of grades awarded is plotted and a comparison of the frequency distributions between markers is assessed for variance)
    · a random blind review process where groups of assignments/ submissions are double-marked and the results compared (Webb et al 2003).

The objective of the moderation process is both to review grades and refine the assessment or marking schema to maximise reliability between the different assessors. There is a degree of professional judgement involved in any assessment process. It is, however, important for those people grading the portfolios to ensure that they share a clear understanding of the aims of the portfolio and assessment criteria. In addition, as much as possible of this information needs to be communicated to the student and/or applicant.

By now you will recognise that portfolios have a place in the assessment of learning as part of educational programmes, organisational performance reviews and individual career planning. The assessment of a portfolio is clearly linked to the portfolio purpose, regardless of whether the portfolio is for an individual seeking to enact a career pathway or an educator, regulator or employer using portfolios to stimulate learning and make judgements about individual suitability. We have discussed the relevance of incremental merit-based grades and criterion-referenced assessment, and applied these to grading rubrics and checklists. Integral to the message of this chapter is the responsibility of the assessor to design assessment processes that positively influence learning outcomes and are fair.

The information covered in this chapter is reinforced by the following comments from Jean Gilmour, an experienced assessor of portfolios across academic and regulatory contexts.

Practice exemplar

Jean Gilmour, a senior lecturer in the School of Health Sciences at Massey University (New Zealand), has been involved in assessing the nurse practitioner applicants. Jean has provided the following practice exemplar:

Assessing portfolios is a complex task. Therefore, think carefully about how best to communicate effectively your competence and professional contributions to the portfolio reviewer. A scholarly, fit-for-purpose and well-structured portfolio is a powerful communication tool for showcasing your practice and your ability.

Some specific strategies to consider when developing a portfolio are as follows:

· Gather evidence as the opportunities arise, even if you are not planning on applying for an advanced practice role. Aspirations change and grow as your career progresses. Substantial evidence developed over a sustained time period is required to demonstrate practice at advanced levels.
· Maintain confidentiality when developing case studies and including referral letters and similar documentation. If the people you have cared for can be identified and there is no evidence of consent for the purpose the information is being used for, questions will be raised in terms of professional conduct.
· Take the time to review relevant standards/competencies carefully and make sure you understand the level/scope of practice required to meet them. Producing evidence demonstrating a less advanced stage of practice will disadvantage you.
· Make sure your evidence is clearly linked to the relevant competency. Do not put the reviewer in the position of having to guess why a piece of evidence might have been included.
· Engage in peer-review processes and mentoring arrangements with your colleagues during portfolio development. Critique of your evidence will challenge your assumptions and expand your practice horizons.
· Take care to demonstrate that your practice is culturally safe, a requirement in the New Zealand nursing and midwifery context. Evidence of cultural safety includes demonstrating your ability to be

reflexive about the values and practices of your own culture and health service culture, along with the impact of those values and practices on the options and perceptions of the people using the health services. Case studies and practice accounts illustrating culturally safe practice, verified by an appropriate person such as the person receiving care and/or a culturally appropriate third party, are important sources of evidence.

Summary points

· Portfolios can be used to support learning and assess any number of outcomes that align with personal and professional self determination.
· The purpose of awarding grades is to communicate achievements succinctly.
· Grades awarded to portfolios may be incremental merit-based grades (e.g. pass through to distinction), criterion-referenced grades (e.g. pass/fail) or a combination of both using assessment hurdles within incremental merit-based grading system.
· The grading approach used should reflect the purpose of the assessment.
· Scoring rubrics are increasingly being used by assessors to grade complex tasks such as portfolios.
· Feedback needs to support the intent of the assessment, namely to provide incentive and skills for further learning, and/or to understand the basis of the achievement being recognised.
· Collaboration between team members and other assessors is required to support valid (assess what is being intended) and reliable (consistently applied) assessment.

Conclusion

This chapter has provided an overview of practices and principles related to portfolio assessment to support the development of quality practice. It has been long understood that student learning is driven by assessment. Students are rewarded by grades and recognition, and as a consequence engage with learning tasks when the relationship between these tasks and their assessment is apparent. To achieve intended learning, however, assessments need to be designed in a manner that supports the achievement of the quality learning outcomes. Assessment guidelines and requirements that are confusing, overly laden with technological or other distractors or do not relate to the students' perceptions of 'real world practice' can result in negative learning. In these scenarios, students might fail to learn and develop the skills that were intended, or possibly worse, develop negative attitudes to learning and change. In addition to providing assignment instructions that are clear and are associated with supportive learning resources, assessment feedback schemas need to also support intended learning outcomes. Assessment grading and feedback should be a transparent exercise, whereby the learner is provided with sufficient information and incentive to allow them to understand what is required to achieve a superior product. Increasingly, assessment feedback schemas and rubrics are routinely provided as part of the assignment instructions. Importantly, students and others submitting their work to be assessed need to understand what these schemas mean in order benefit from this information. This chapter has provided this level of information, so that the rationales and approaches within assessment design and implementation can be understood by all participants in the assessment process.

References

André, K., 2000. 'Grading student clinical practice performance: the Australian perspective'. Nurse Education Today 20 (8), 672—679.

André, K., 2002. The assessment of undergraduate clinical performance: the communication of nursing. School of Nursing and Midwifery, Faculty of Health Sciences, Flinders University, Adelaide.

Andre, K., 2010. E-Portfolios for the aspiring professional, Collegian: Journal of the Royal College of Nursing Australia 17 (3), 119—124.

André, K., van Eck, D., 2010. School of Nursing and Midwifery Step 2010 final report. University of South Australia, Adelaide.

André, K., Heartfield, M., 2007. Professional portfolios: evidence of competency for nurses and midwives. Elsevier, Marrickville, NSW.

Andrews, R., 2010. Argumentation in Higher Education: improving practice through theory and research. Routledge, New York.

Australian Commission on Safety and Quality in Healthcare, 2006. Background information and resources section of the measurement for improvement toolkit Commonwealth of Australia Accessed online 15 October 2010 at: http://www.safetyandquality.gov.au/internet/safety/publishing.nsf/Content/703C98BF37524DFDCA25729600128BD2/$File/Toolkit_PartB.pdf.

Australian ePortfolio Project, ePortfolio use by university students in Australia, 2008. Developing a sustainable community of practice, Stage 1 Final project report. August 2008 Accessed online 7 January 2010 at: http://www.eportfoliopractice.qut.edu.au/docs/Aep_Final_Report/AeP_Report_ebook.pdf.

Australian ePortfolio Project, ePortfolio use by university students in Australia, 2009. Developing a sustainable community of practice, Stage 2 Final project report: December 2009. Accessed online June 2010 at: http://www.eportfoliopractice.qut.edu.au/information2/report_stage2/index.jsp.

Australian Flexible Learning Framework, 2009. E-portfolios for RPL assessment. Department of Education Employment and Workplace Relations, Canberra.

Australian Health Practitioner Regulation Agency, 2009. Health Practitioner Regulation National Law Act 2009 Accessed online 15 November 2010 at: http://www.ahpra.gov.au/.

Australian Institute of Health and Welfare, 2010. International information on the safety and quality of health care. Accessed online 19 October 2010 at: http://www.aihw.gov.au/safequalityhealth/international_stats.cfm.

Australian Nursing Council, 2002. Principles for the Assessment of National Competency Standards for Registered and Enrolled Nurses, Canberra, 1—11.

Australian Nursing and Midwifery Council, 2007. Development of a national framework for the demonstration of continuing competence for nurses and midwives — literature review. Australian Nursing and Midwifery Council, Canberra.

Australian Nursing and Midwifery Council, 2007. National framework for the development of decision-making tools for nursing and midwifery practice. Accessed online 12 December 2010 at: http://www.nursingmidwiferyboard.gov.au/Codes-and-Guidelines.aspx.

Australian Nursing and Midwifery Council, 2008a. National Competency Standards for the Registered Nurse. Accessed online 19 January 2011 at: http://www.nursingmidwiferyboard.gov.au/Codes-and-Guidelines.aspx

Australian Nursing and Midwifery Council, 2008b. National Competency Standards for the Midwife. Accessed online 10 August 2010 at: http://www.nursingmidwiferyboard.gov.au/documents/default.aspx?record=WD10%2f1350&dbid=AP&chksum=Yp0233q3xmE5YVjiy%2fy0mA%3d%3d.

Australian Nursing and Midwifery Council, 2008c. Code of Professional Conduct for Nurses in Australia. Accessed online 10 August 2010 at: http://www.nursingmidwiferyboard.gov.au/documents/default.aspx?record=WD10%2f1353&dbid=AP&chksum=Ac7KxRPDt289C5Bx%2ff4q3Q%3d%3d.

Australian Nursing and Midwifery Council, 2008d. Code of Professional Conduct for Midwives in Australia. Accessed online 10 August 2010 at: http://www.nursingmidwiferyboard.gov.au/documents/default.aspx?record=WD10%2f1355&dbid=AP&chksum=Mm624fvql2ZEKdEmT3l2ng%3d%3d.

Australian Nursing and Midwifery Council, 2008e. Code of Ethics for Nurses in Australia, August 2008. Accessed online 19 January 2011 at: http://www.nursingmidwiferyboard.gov.au/documents/default.aspx?record=WD10%2f1352&dbid=AP&chksum=GTNolhwLC8lnBn7hiEFeag%3d%3d.

Baptiste, S., 2005. Changing face of entry to occupational therapy practice: some personal reflections from a person environment occupation perspective. Australian Occupational Therapy Journal 52 (3), 179.

Barrett, H., 2007. Researching electronic portfolios and learner engagement: the REFLECT initiative. Journal of Adolescent and Adult Literacy 50 (6), 436–449.

Barrett, H., 2009. Balancing the two faces of ePortfolios. Accessed online 15 September 2010 at: http://electronicportfolios.org/balance/index.html.

Barrett, H., 2010. Balancing the two faces of ePortfolios. Accessed online 23 November 2010 at: http://eft.educom.pt/index.php/eft/article/viewFile/161/102.

Barrie, S., Hughes, C., Smith, C., 2009. The national graduate attributes project: integration and assessment of graduate attributes in curriculum. Australian Learning and Teaching Council, Strawberry Hill, NSW.

Benner, P., 1984. From novice to expert: excellence and power in clinical nursing practice. Addison-Wesley, Menlo Park, CA.

Benner, P., Sutphen, M., Leonard, V., Day, L., 2010. Educating nurses: a call for radical transformation. Jossey-Bass, San Francisco, CA.

Best, R., Best, R., 2009. The use of assessment hurdles: pedagogy v. practicality. Paper presented at the 34th Australasian Universities Building Educators Conference (AUBEA 2009), Barossa Valley, South Australia.

Biggs, J., Tang, C., 2007. Teaching for quality learning at university. Society for Research into Higher Education and Open University Press, Buckingham.

Billett, S., 2006. Learning practice: conceptualising professional lifelong learning. University of Leeds, Leeds.

Boreham, N., 2004. Collective competence and work process knowledge. Paper presented at the Symposium on Work Process Knowledge in European, Vocational Education and Training Research, European Conference on Educational Research. University of Crete, Greece. September 2004.

Boreham, N., Shea, C., Mackway-Jones, K., 2000. Clinical risk and collective competence in the hospital emergency department in the UK. Social Science and Medicine 51 (1), 83–91.

Bondy, K., 1983. "Criterion-referenced definitions for rating scales in clinical evaluation." Journal of Nurse Education 22 (9), 376—382.

Boud, D., Falchikov, N., 2006. Aligning assessment with long-term learning. Assessment and Evaluation in Higher Education 31 (4), 399—413.

Boud, D., Solomon, N., 2001. Work-based learning — a new higher education? Open University Press, Philadelphia.

Boud, D., Keough, R., Walker, D., 1985. Reflection: turning experience into learning. Kogan, London.

Branch, W.T., Paranjape, A., 2002. Feedback and reflection: teaching methods for clinical settings. Academic Medicine 77 (12), 1185—1188.

Briant, R., Schug, S., Scott, A., et al., 2001. Adverse events in New Zealand public hospitals: principal findings from a national survey. Ministry of Health, Wellington, New Zealand. Accessed online 1 October 2010 at: http://www.moh.govt.nz/publications/adverseevents.

Bryant, R., 2005. Issue paper. Regulation, roles and competency development. International Council of Nurses, Geneva.

Bryne, M., Schroeter, K., Carter, S., Mower, J., 2009. The professional portfolio: an evidence-based assessment method. Journal of Continuing Education in Nursing 40 (12), 545—552.

Bulman, C., 2008a. Help to get you started. In: Bulman, C., Schutz, S. (Eds.), Reflective practice in nursing. Blackwell, Chichester, UK, pp. 219—239.

Bulman, C., 2008b. An introduction to reflection. In: Bulman, C., Schutz, S. (Eds.), Reflective practice in nursing. Blackwell, Chichester, UK, pp. 1—24.

Bulman, C., Schutz, S. (Eds.), 2008. Reflective practice in nursing. Blackwell, Chichester, UK.

Campbell, D., Melenyzer, B., Nettles, D., Wyman, R., 2000. Portfolio and performance assessment in teacher education. Allyn & Bacon, Needham Heights.

Clouder, L., Sellars, J., 2004. Reflective practice and clinical supervision: an interprofessional perspective. Journal of Advanced Nursing 46 (3), 262—269.

Commonwealth of Australia 2005. Australia's health workforce. Productivity Commission Research Report, Canberra.

Cooper, T., Emden, C., 2001. Portfolio assessment: a guide for nurses and midwives. Praxis Education, Western Australia.

Curtis, K., 2005. The importance of self-regulation in the implementation of data protection principles: The Australian private sector experience. Australian Government Office of Privacy Commissioner, Montreux.

Donner, G., Wheeler, M., 2004. Taking control of your nursing career. Elsevier, Sydney.

EdCaN, 2008. Competency assessment in nursing: a summary of literature published since 2000. Report prepared on behalf of National Education Framework for Cancer Nursing (EDCaN) by Alison Evans Consulting. Accessed online 19 January 2011 at: http://www.edcan.org/pdf/EdCancompetenciesliteraturereviewFINAL.pdf.

Egan, R., Testa, D., 2010. Models of supervision. In: Stagnitti, K., Schoo, A., Welch, D. (Eds.), Clinical and fieldwork placement in the health professions. Oxford University Press, Melbourne, pp. 145—158.

Emden, C., Hutt, D., Bruce, M., 2003. Portfolio learning/assessment in nursing and midwifery: an innovation in progress. Contemporary Nurse 16 (1-2), 124—132.

Eraut, M., 2003. Developing professional knowledge and competence. Falmer Press, London.

Eva, K.W., 2004. On the generality of specificity. Medical Education 37, 587—588.

Evans, M., Powell, A., 2007. Conceptual and practical issues related to the design for sustainability of communities of practice: the case of e-portfolio use in pre-service teacher training. Technology. Pedagogy and Education 16 (2), 199—214.

Ewell, P., 2008. Assessment and accountability in America today: background and context. New Directions for Institutional Research. Assessment Supplement 2008, 7—16.

Gaberson, K., Oermann, M.H. (Eds.), 2007. Clinical teaching strategies in nursing. Springer, New York.

Gibbs, G., Farmer, B., Eastcott, D., 1988. Learning by doing: a guide to teaching and learning methods. Further Education Unit, Oxford Polytechnic, Oxford.

Glasgow, N., Wells, R., Butler, J., et al., 2006. Using competency-based education to equip the primary health care workforce to manage chronic disease. September 2006. Australian Primary Health Care Research Institute (APHCRI), ANU College of Medicine and Health Sciences. Australian National University, Canberra.

Green, M., Reddy, S., Holmboe, E., 2009. Teaching and evaluating point of care learning with an internet-based clinical-question portfolio. Journal of Continuing Education in the Health Professions 29 (4), 209—219.

Haines, C., Scott, K., Lincoln, R. for Miles Morgan Australia Pty Ltd 2006 Australian blueprint for career development (draft prototype). Career Development Section, Enterprise and Career Development Branch, Department of Education, Science and Training, Commonwealth of Australia, Canberra.

Hayes, L.J., Orchard, C., McGillis Hall, L., et al., 2006. Career intentions of nursing students and new nurse graduates: a review of the literature. International Journal of Nursing Education Scholarship 3 (1) Article 26.

Health Practitioner Regulation National Law Act, 2009. Accessed online 1st October 2010 at http://www.ahpra.gov.au/Legislation-and-Publications/Legislation.aspx.

Heartfield, 2006. National Nursing and Nursing Education Taskforce 2005, p 38.

Huang, T., Liang, S., 2005. A randomized clinical trial of the effectiveness of discharging intervention in hospitalized elders with hip fracture due to falling. Journal of Clinical Nursing 14 (10), 1193—1201.

Hull, C., Redfern, L., Shuttleworth, A., 2005. Profiles and portfolios: a guide for health and social care. Palgrave Macmillan, London.

International Council of Nurses, 2001. It's your career: take charge career planning and development. International Council of Nurses, Geneva.

Jasper, M., 2006. Professional development, reflection and decision-making. Blackwell Publishing, Oxford, UK.

Jasper, M., Fulton, J., 2005. Marking criteria for assessing practice-based portfolios at masters' level. Nurse Education Today 25, 377—389.

Joyes, G., Gray, L., Hartnell-Young, E., 2010. Effective practice with e-portfolios: how can the UK experience inform implementation? Australasian Journal of Educational Technology 26 (1), 15—27.

Kanter, R.M., 1989. Careers and the wealth of nations: a macro-perspective on the structure and implications of career forms. In: Arthur, M.B., Hall, D.T., Lawrence, B. (Eds.), Handbook of career theory. Cambridge University Press, Cambridge.

Kingma, M., 2006. Nurses on the Move Migration and the Global Health Care Economy. Cornell University Press, New York.

Knowles, M., 1984. Andragogy in action: applying modern principles of adult education. Jossey-Bass, San Francisco.

Karlowicz, K., 2010. Development and testing of a portfolio evaluation scoring tool. Journal of Nursing Education 49 (2), 78—86.

Kitchener, K.S., King, P.M., De Luca, S., 2006. Development of reflective judgment in adulthood. In: Hoare, C. (Ed.), Handbook of adult development and learning. Oxford University Press, New York, pp. 73—98.

Kolb, D., 1984. Experiential learning: experience as the source of learning and development. Prentice-Hall, Englewood Cliffs, NJ.

Liamputtong, P., Ezzy, D., 2005. Qualitative Research Methods. Oxford University Press, Melbourne, Victoria.

MacKenzie, C., 2004. The politics of representation: a personal reflection on the problematic positioning of the midwifery educator. Studies in Continuing Education 26 (1), 117—127.

Mertler, C., 2001. "Designing Scoring Rubrics for your Classroom". Practical Assessment, Research & Evaluation 7 (25). Accessed June 2010 http://PAREonline.net/getvn.asp?v=7&n=25.

McMullan, M., Endacott, Gray, M., Miller, C., Scholes, J., Webb, C., 2003. Portfolios and assessment of competence: a review of the literature. Journal of Advanced Nursing 41 (3), 283—294.

Midwifery Council of New Zealand, 2008. Competencies for Entry to the Register. Retrieved 8th September, 2009, from http://www.midwiferycouncil.org.nz/content/library/Competencies_for_Entry_to_the_Register1.pdf.

Midwifery Council of New Zealand, 2008. Midwifery Council of New Zealand recertification programme: competence-based practising certificates for midwives. Policy document. Accessed online 19 October 2010 at: http://www.nursingcouncil.org.nz/download/115/framework-pdrp-jun08.pdf.

Monash University, 2010. Sample critical incident report. Accessed online 13 September 2010 at: http://www.monash.edu.au/lls/llonline/writing/medicine/reflective/5.xml.

National Health and Medical Research Council, Department of Health and Ageing, 2004. The impact of privacy legislation on NHMRC stakeholders: comparative stakeholder analysis. Accessed online 3 December 2010 at: http://www.nhmrc.gov.au/_files_nhmrc/file/about/st8.pdf.

National Health Workforce Taskforce, April 2009. Health workforce in Australia and factors influencing current shortages. Accessed online 19 October 2010 at: http://www.ahwo.gov.au/publications.asp.

National Nursing Organisations Members and Links Members of the Coalition and Associates, 2006. National Nursing Organisations Secretariat. Australian Nursing Federation Head Office, Canberra.

Norman, K., 2008. Providing evidence of achievement. In: Norman, K. (Ed.), Portfolios in the nursing profession. Quay Books, London.

Nursing and Midwifery Board of Australia, 2006. Accessed online 25 November 2010 at: http://www.nursingmidwiferyboard.gov.au/.

Nursing and Midwifery Board of Australia, 2010. Continuing professional development registration standard. Accessed online 1 November 2010 at: http://www.nursingmidwiferyboard.gov.au/Registration-Standards.aspx.

Nursing Council of New Zealand, 2005a. New Zealand Health Practitioners Competence Assurance Act. Accessed online 21 November 2010 at: http://www.nursingcouncil.org.nz.

Nursing Council of New Zealand, 2005b. Competencies for the nurse assistant and enrolled nurse: scopes of practice. Nursing Council of New Zealand, Wellington.

Nursing Council of New Zealand, 2008. Competencies for Nurse Practitioners. Accessed online 3 December 2010 at: http://www.nursingcouncil.org.nz/download/119/np-competencies-dec-08.pdf.

Nursing Council of New Zealand, 2008. Nurse Practitioner Endorsement — guidelines for applicants. from http://www.nursingcouncil.org.nz/npracguidelinessep02.pdf.

Nursing Council of New Zealand, 2010. Guideline. Expanded practice for registered nurses. September 2010. Accessed online 21 November 2010 at: http://www.nursingcouncil.org.nz.

Office of the Australian Information Commissioner. About Privacy. Accessed online 4 December 2010 at: http://www.privacy.gov.au/aboutprivacy.

Pairman, S., 2005. From autonomy and back again: educating midwives across a century: part 1. New Zealand College of Midwives Journal 33, 6—11.

Paley, J., 2006. Evidence and expertise. Nursing Inquiry 13 (2), 82—93.

Palmer, A., Burns, S., Bulman, C. (Eds.), 1994. Reflective practice in nursing. Blackwell Scientific Publications, Oxford.

Pearce, R., 2003. Profiles and Portfolios of Evidence. Nelson Thornes, Cheltenham, UK.

Price, K., Heartfield, M., Gibson, T., 2001. Nursing career pathways. National Nursing Education Review, Department of Education. Training and Youth Affairs, Canberra.

Quinn, F.M., Hughes, S.J., 2007. Quinn's principles and practice of nurse education. Nelson Thornes, Cheltenham, UK.

Rafferty, A., Ball, J., Aiken, L., 2001. Are Teamwork and Professional Autonomy Compatible, and Do They Result in Improved Hospital Care? Quality in Health Care 10, 32—37.

Reeves, S., Zwarenstein, M., Goldman, J., et al., 2008. Interprofessional education: effects on professional practice and health care outcomes. Cochrane Database of Systematic Reviews (issue 1) art. no.: CD002213. DOI: 10.1002/14651858.CD002213.pub2. Accessed online 14 October 2010 at: http://www2.cochrane.org/reviews/en/ab002213.html.

Riley, R., Manias, E., 2004. The uses of photography in clinical nursing practice and research: a literature review. Journal of Advanced Nursing 48 (4), 397—405.

Roberts, C., O'Rouke, A., 2002. Portfolio-based assessments in medical education: are they reliable and valid for summative purposes? Medical Education 36, 899—900.

Royal College of Nursing Australia, 2006. 3LP Life long learning program. from http://www.rcna.org.au/pages/3lp.php.

Russell, L., 2010. Analysis of the 2010—2011 health and ageing budget. Menzies Centre for Health Policy, University of Sydney/Australian National University. Accessed online 15 October 2010 at: http://www.menzieshealthpolicy.edu.au/other_tops/pdfs_pubs/2010-11budgetanalysis.pdf.

Sackley, C.M., Pound, K., 2002. Stroke patients entering nursing home care: a content analysis of discharge letters. Clinical Rehabilation 16 (7), 736—740.

Santy, J., Smith, L., 2007. Being an e-learner in health and social care: a students guide. Routledge, New York.

Sackett, D., Strauss, S., Richardson, W., et al., 2000. Evidence based medicine: how to practice and teach EBM. Churchill Livingstone, London.

Scholes, J., Webb, J., Gray, M., et al., 2004. Making portfolios work in practice. Journal of Advanced Nursing 46 (6), 595—603.

Schön, D., 1983. The reflective practitioner: how professionals think in action. Basic Books, New York.

Schön, D., 1987. Educating the reflective practitioner. Jossey-Bass, San Francisco, CA.

Schuster, P.M., 2008. Concept mapping: a critical thinking approach to care planning. FA Davis, Philadelphia, PA.

Smee, S., 2003. Skill based assessment. British Medical Journal 362, 703—706.

Spence, W., 2004. Portfolio assessment: practice teachers' early experience. Nurse Education Today 24, 388—401.

Stefani, L., Mason, R., Pegler, C., 2007. The educational potential of e-portfolios: supporting personal development and reflective learning. Routledge, London.

Storey, L., Haigh, C., 2002. Portfolios in professional practice. Nurse Education in Practice 2, 44—48.

Stuart, C., 2004. The use of portfolios in clinical evidence to influence student learning in midwifery education. Birth Issues 13 (4), 121—127.

Taylor, B., 2006. Reflective practice: a guide for nurses and midwives. Open University Press, London.

Taylor, B., 2006. Reflective practice: a guide for nurses and midwives. Open University Press, London.

Thomson, C., 2004. The regulation of health information privacy in Australia. National Health and Medical Research Council. Accessed online 6 December 2010 at: http://www.nhmrc.gov.au/_files_nhmrc/file/publications/synopses/nh53.pdf.

Wang, H., 2004. 'Involve me, I will understand': how to improve students' understanding in the mathematics course ordinary differential equations. China Papers November 2004, 64—67.

Ward, A., Gracey, J., 2006. Reflective practice in physiotherapy curricula: a survey of UK university-based professional practice coordinators. Medical Teacher 28 (1), 32—39.

Washington State University, 2009. Evolution of our eportfolio thinking. Accessed online June 2009 at: https://teamsite.oue.wsu.edu/progeval/eport/evolution/default.aspx.

Webb, C., Endacott, R., 2002. Commentries: Models of Portfolios. Medical Education 36, 897—898.

Webb, C., Endacott, R., Gray, M., et al., 2003. Evaluating portfolio assessment systems: what are the appropriate criteria? Nurse Education Today 23, 600—609.

Glossary

Australian Health Practitioner Regulation Agency (AHPRA): This organisation is responsible for the implementation of the National Registration and Accreditation Scheme across Australia through the various National Health Practitioner Boards. These Boards include the Nursing and Midwifery Board of Australia and their role is to protect the public and set standards and policies that all registered health practitioners must meet.

Australian Nursing and Midwifery Accreditation Council (ANMAC): This authority has replaced the Australian Nursing and Midwifery Council (ANMC). It is the independent **accrediting** authority for nursing and midwifery under the National Registration and Accreditation Scheme. It sets standards for accreditation and accredits nursing and midwifery courses and providers.

Assessment: A systematic procedure for collecting qualitative and quantitative data to describe progress and ascertain deviations from expected outcomes and achievements (NCNZ 2005).

Authorisation: The process through which nursing and midwifery regulatory authorities sanction the practice of nurse practitioners within their jurisdiction. The authorisation process invests legal authority and responsibilities on the person so authorised. Once an applicant is authorised, he or she will be registered (i.e. have his or her details entered on a written record) and the nursing and midwifery regulatory authority will endorse (i.e. openly approve of) his or her practice as a nurse practitioner.

Autonomy: Having a sense of one's own identity and an ability to act independently and to exert control over one's environment, including a sense of task mastery, internal locus of control, and self-efficacy.

Attributes: Characteristics that underpin competent performance (ANMC 2005).

Client/patient: A person or persons who engage(s) or is/are served by the professional advice or services of another. May refer to an individual, family or community. Use of 'client' acknowledges that a significant proportion of nursing services are delivered to people who are well and proactively engaging in healthcare. Use of 'patient' acknowledges that nursing provides some of its services to people who are sick and, in the true Latin meaning, are 'suffering'. However, 'client' and 'patient' are used synonymously to acknowledge that the same services may be used for both clients and patients.

Competence: The combination of skills, knowledge, attitudes, values and abilities that underpin effective and/or superior performance in a profession/occupational area (ANMC 2005).

Competent: The person has competence across all the domains of competencies applicable to the nurse, at a standard that is judged to be appropriate for the level of nurse being assessed (ANMC 2005, NCNZ 2005).

Competency standards: Consist of competency units and competency elements (ANMC 2005).

Context: The setting/environment where competence can be demonstrated or applied (ANMC 2005, NCNZ 2005).

Cues/indicators: Key generic examples of competent performance. They are neither comprehensive nor exhaustive. They assist the assessor when using their professional judgement in assessing nursing practice. They further assist curriculum development (ANMC 2005, NCNZ 2005).

Enrolled nurse: i) A person licensed under an Australian state or territory nurses act or health professionals act to provide nursing care under the supervision of a registered nurse. Referred to as a registered nurse division II in Victoria (ANMC 2005); ii) A nurse registered under the *enrolled nurse* scope of practice (NCNZ 2005).

ePortfolios: Use of online or electronic technologies to achieve the same aims as other forms of portfolio.

Evidence: Objective and subjective information that forms the basis of a portfolio. Portfolio evidence may take different forms including objects, statements, documents, recordings and other products that demonstrate and support the achievements and claims.

Exemplars: Concrete, key examples chosen to be typical of competence. They are not the standard but are indicative of the standard (ANMC 2005).

Indicators: *See 'Cues'*

Lifelong learning: A full and successful life including effective work performance requires continued openness to, and participation in, education and learning. This learning may take place through a range of sources from university and vocational formal qualifications to other types of programs, courses and events, as well as on-the-job training and personal and informal learning.

Nurse practitioner: Like the nurse and the midwife, this is a person who is educated and authorised by the necessary authorities and specifically registered in the scope of practice for nurse practitioner (ANMC 2006), (Nursing Council of New Zealand 2008). The nurse practitioner has particular responsibilities to perform autonomously and collaboratively in an advanced and extended clinical role.

Nursing Council of New Zealand (NCNZ): The responsible authority for nurses in New Zealand with legislated functions under the *Health Practitioners Competence Assurance Act 2003*. The NCNZ governs the practice of nurses by setting and monitoring standards of registration, which ensures safe and competent care for the public of New Zealand. As the statutory authority, the NCNZ is committed to enhancing professional excellence in nursing (NCNZ 2005).

Patient: *See 'Client'*

Performance assessment: Measurement against professional, educational and/or organisational criteria of how an individual uses their knowledge and skills to produce or complete the required level of performance.

Performance criteria: Descriptive statements that can be assessed and that reflect the intent of a competency in terms of performance, behaviour and circumstance (NCNZ 2005).

Portfolios: Compilation of a portfolio requires purposeful selection and structuring of different types of evidence to meet specific goals. These may include individual professional goals, competencies, career achievements and continuing professional development activities and experiences portfolio may be developed for education, certification, employment or promotion purposes. Depending on the specific purpose, a portfolio may highlight only best practice examples of competency and performance-based achievements, as well as a summative evaluation of strengths and weaknesses, or may also include 'works in progress' that show development and improvement over time.

Reflective practice: A way of learning that involves using personal experience as a basis from which to identify and understand the knowledge that is developed from and used in practice.

Reliability: The extent to which a tool will function consistently in the same way with repeated use (NCNZ 2005).

Scopes of practice: In the context of nursing and midwifery, this term refers to the complete range of roles, functions, responsibilities, activities and decision-making abilities that nurses and midwives are educated, competent and authorised by their regulators and employers to perform.

Validity: The extent to which a measurement tool measures what it purports to measure (NCNZ 2005).

References

Australian Nursing and Midwifery Council (2008a). National Competency Standards for the Registered Nurse. Accessed online 19 January 2011 at: http://www.nursingmidwiferyboard.gov.au.

Australian Nursing and Midwifery Council National competency standards for the nurse practitioner. Nursing and Midwifery Board of Australia Accessed online 3rd December 2010 at http://www.nursingmidwiferyboard.gov.au/Codes-and-Guidelines.aspx.

Nursing Council of New Zealand (2008). Competencies for Nurse Practitioners Accessed online 3rd December 2010 at http://www.nursingcouncil.org.nz/download/119/np-competencies-dec-08.pdf.

Nursing Council of New Zealand (2005). Competencies for the registered nurse: scope of practice. www.nursingcouncil.org.nz/competenciesrn.pdf 29 Jan 2007.

Nursing Council of New Zealand Scopes of practice. Notice of Scopes of Practice and Related Qualifications Prescribed by the Nursing Council of New Zealand Wellington. Online resources available at: http://www.nursingcouncil.org.nz/scopes.html. (Accessed on 7th Feb 2007.)

Index